MW01011662

30-DAY HEALTHY WEIGHT-LOSS PLAN AND COOKBOOK

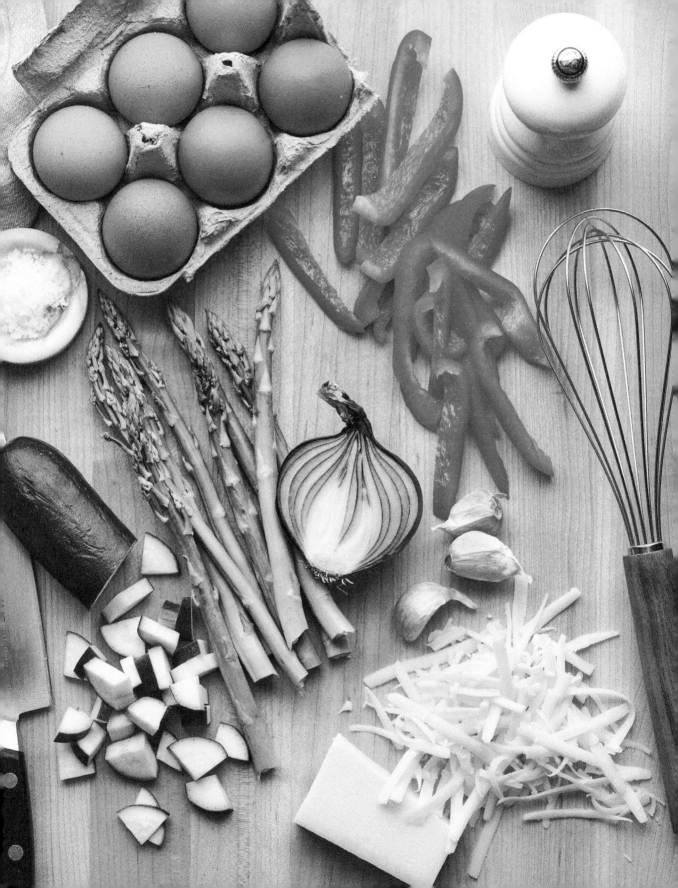

30-DAY HEALTHY WEIGHT-LOSS PLAN AND COOKBOOK

100 Easy Recipes and Workouts for a Balanced Life

Kelli Shallal, MPH, RD, CPT, CLT

Photography by Andrew Purcell

ROCKRIDGE
PRESS

Interior and Cover Designer: Amanda Kirk
Art Producer: Meg Baggott
Editor: Laura Apperson
Associate Editor: Maxine Marshall
Production Editor: Emily Sheehan
Photography © 2020 Andrew Purcell.
Food styling by Carrie Purcell.
Illustrations © 2020 Mat Edwards
Author photo courtesy of Nerissa Lowicki

ISBN: Print 978-1-64739-752-4
eBook 978-1-64739-453-0
R0

To my family, for always supporting my dreams and trying my recipes. And to the victims and their families who lost their lives, jobs, or well-being due to COVID-19, my heart and prayers are with you.

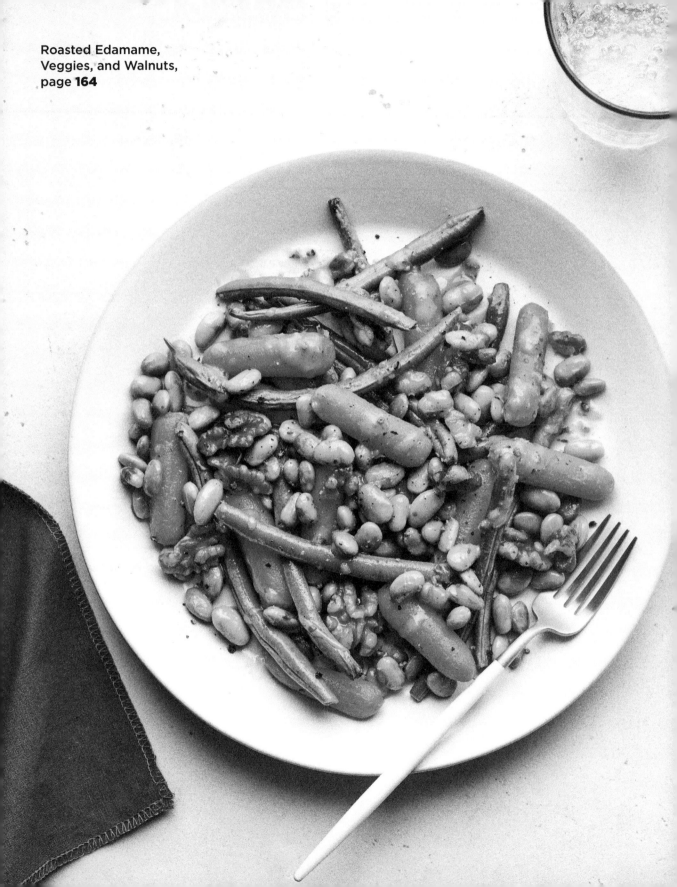

Roasted Edamame,
Veggies, and Walnuts,
page **164**

CONTENTS

INTRODUCTION

I was raised in the 1990s, and growing up, I ate either Southern fried food drenched in butter and cooked by my grandma or run-of-the-mill processed food. I distinctly remember coming home from college and asking my grandma to make cauliflower soup. She was confused, so I described it as cauliflower, butter, and Velveeta cheese. She laughed and said, "Oh, darling, that's just cauliflower."

I am now a registered dietitian and personal trainer, and I became those things because of how little knowledge I had about nutrition. I spent a long time trying to figure out what good nutrition actually means.

At first, I thought it meant starving yourself of calories and all flavor in your food. I learned the hard way that it isn't a sustainable approach. I counted calories, which naturally led to restricting calories, fat, and carbs. I ate a lot of fake, low-calorie processed foods, and while it worked initially, it then backfired in a major way. My hormones didn't just rebel, they shut down entirely, which made it hard to maintain my weight even at only 1,200 calories a day. I had to do a lot of painstaking work to rebuild my metabolism and rebalance my hormones. If I had taken a more sustainable approach to start with, I would never have had to go through that. I will share this better approach to weight loss with you in chapter 1.

Did you know that the average American starts a diet multiple times a year? I share this fact every chance I get because it shows that diets aren't sustainable. So if diets don't work, what should you do? Most people who want to adopt a healthier lifestyle don't know where to start.

That's what I love about this 30-day weight loss plan. It's all about getting started, and it isn't intended to be a one-and-done. It generates powerful momentum and results that will last well beyond 30 days. This is because while you are following the 30-day plan, you're learning valuable lifestyle skills and habits—including cooking, nutrition, and exercise—that you will take with you beyond the 30 days.

This awesome 30-day program is complete with weekly meal plans and shopping lists to make it as easy as possible for you and to keep life from getting in the way. It also includes simple exercises you can do at home with minimal equipment. And then, of course, there are healthy recipes that use everyday, affordable ingredients, many of which use just five ingredients (not counting the salt, pepper, and cooking oil), use just one pot or pan, are baked on a sheet pan, take just 30 minutes from start to finish, or require no cooking at all. Honestly, that's just how I cook! I may be a foodie/food blogger/dietitian, but I don't have time to spend all day in the kitchen trying to get a healthy dinner that tastes good on the table. If you want to fit healthy eating into your life, then it has to be fast and efficient, or it won't stick.

Luckily, this plan is just that: It's fast, it's efficient, and it gives you all the tools you need to jump-start your healthy lifestyle. Remember what they say: Don't look back in 60 days and wish you had started 30 days ago. Start now! I can't wait to accompany you at the beginning of your journey to optimal health and fitness!

PART ONE

WELCOME TO A HEALTHIER YOU

Congrats on committing to a healthier you! Sometimes, we need a jump-start to get us going on the right track. This book will not only be your guide to a healthier you but will also give you the road map to help you reach your goals. Let's dive in!

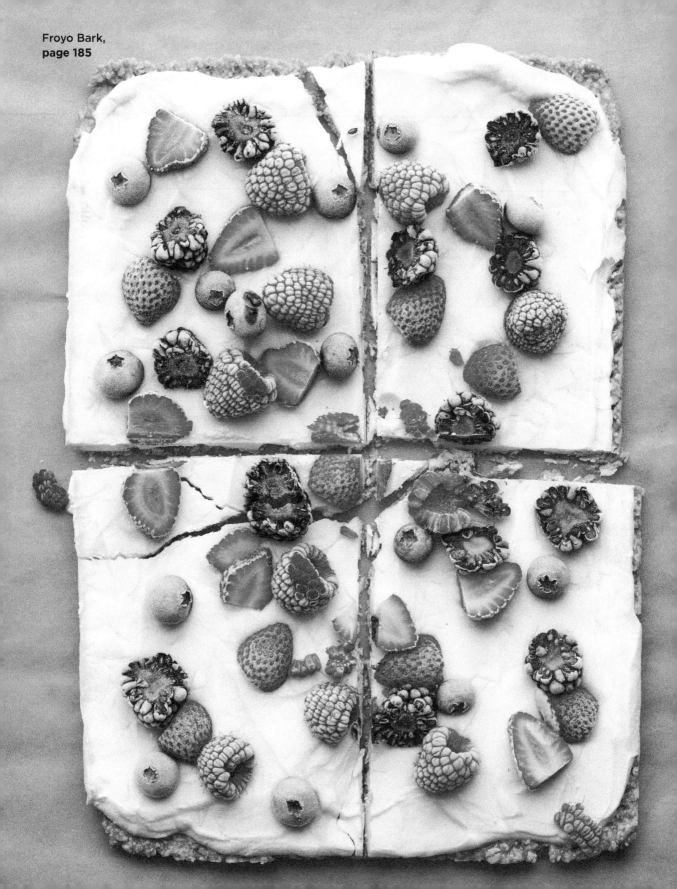

Froyo Bark,
page 185

CHAPTER 1

A Healthy Approach to Losing Weight

IT'S NO SECRET THAT THE STANDARD AMERICAN DIET IS composed of mostly low-nutrient, calorie-dense foods such as refined flours, added sugar, excess preservatives, and addictive flavor enhancers. These foods, although they provide calories, offer us very little in the way of actual nutrition. So even when we aren't hungry, our body lacks nutrients and begins to crave more energy-dense foods. In response, we keep giving it more of the same empty-calorie foods meal after meal after meal, feeding the cycle of endless cravings.

You may feel confused about what is healthy in today's environment of infinite fad diets and changing nutrition research. However, there are some consistencies across populations and dietary patterns that remain true and unchanging and help us define a healthy diet.

In contrast to the standard American diet, a diet full of well-balanced, nutrient-dense foods, including high-fiber carbohydrates, healthy fats, and lean proteins, leaves you feeling both satisfied and energized. Happily, we have taken a giant step in the right direction by realizing that "real food" not only is nutrient-dense but also leaves out questionable food additives and addictive flavor enhancers.

But to get your diet back on track and give yourself a healthy reboot, you need to focus not only on the quality of food you eat (a.k.a. "real food") but also on how to balance those foods on your plate for optimal energy, digestion, and body composition. In this book, you'll learn how to balance your plate, whether you are the one cooking or not.

Ultimately, the goal with this 30-day plan is to jump-start a lifestyle of healthy, balanced eating. Adopting a healthy lifestyle has so many awesome benefits that once you start, you won't want to stop! I've listed just a few of them here.

Lose weight: When you switch to a more balanced way of eating, the foods you eat will keep you feeling full and satisfied, leading to sustainable, long-lasting weight loss—the kind that's easy to maintain! A healthy approach to losing weight is the only sustainable option for improving your health long-term.

Have more energy: Many foods give us calories, but not all of them energize us. Balanced eating means you are choosing more filling, high-quality, nutrient-dense carbohydrates in balanced quantities throughout the day. Eating this way creates stable blood sugar levels, leading to higher energy levels. Losing weight also decreases inflammation levels and demands on your body for energy, meaning you'll have more energy reserves to do the things you love.

Clear out toxins: Contrary to what some diets want you to believe, your body does an excellent job of getting rid of toxins on its own. However, if you are constantly exposing it to toxins and nonnutritive chemicals, your liver will have to work overtime to process all that junk. By choosing healthier, less processed foods, you limit the number of toxins you consume and give your body a chance to clean up without overloading it with more toxins.

Reset metabolism: Here is the big bonus: When you eat enough of the right foods, it fuels your metabolism instead of damaging it. While you do need to be in a calorie deficit to lose weight, if you've been in too low of a calorie deficit for too long, it can hurt your metabolism. In this book, you'll learn how to find the appropriate number of calories for weight loss and weight maintenance to support your metabolism instead of damaging it.

Reduce inflammation: When you adopt a healthy lifestyle, eat fewer processed foods, and lose weight, you decrease inflammation, which is created by excess chemicals, food additives, sugars, and highly processed oils. Chronic inflammation is the underlying root cause of many chronic diseases, including diabetes, cancer, cardiovascular disease, and irritable bowel disease, so by focusing on reducing inflammation and staying healthy, you decrease your risk of developing chronic conditions that you may be genetically inclined to develop. You can also help lessen the severity of symptoms of some conditions you've already developed. For instance, just a 10 percent decrease in overall body weight is shown to improve insulin sensitivity in people with type 2 diabetes and improve blood pressure numbers.

Improve digestion: It's estimated that more than 42 million Americans struggle with constipation, according to the National Institute of Diabetes and Digestive and Kidney Diseases. Eating a healthy, fiber-rich diet will keep you regular, and improved digestion helps you absorb more nutrients and generally feel more comfortable throughout the day. Plus, fiber also helps lower the risk of certain chronic diseases such as colon cancer and cardiovascular disease.

Your weight loss journey is about to begin. *You* define the journey and the experiences within it, and with this knowledge you are about to achieve all your health goals and more!

A Positive Approach to Healthy Eating

For weight loss to be successful long-term, adopt a positive attitude toward your body and healthy eating. Taking a positive approach allows for imperfection. Social gatherings and the food that surrounds them are a part of our lives, and you should not have to avoid them in the quest to live healthier. I can't stress this enough: It's *not* all or nothing.

Even as a dietitian, it took me a long time to understand what balance truly means and to let go of some of my emotions surrounding food. Yes, weight loss requires cleaner eating than weight maintenance, since you're taking into account a necessary calorie deficit, but not so much that you have to lock yourself down and be unable to enjoy any social gatherings. Instead, adopt the attitude that you can have it all—just not all at once.

IT'S NOT ALL OR NOTHING

A positive approach to healthy eating includes understanding that having treats does not make you a bad person. Having a treat or an off-track meal doesn't even mean you slipped up; it's just one meal. In the scheme of three meals a day, 21 meals a week, plus snacks, it doesn't matter at all unless you hyper-focus on it and make it matter.

I see people who want to lose weight self-sabotage over and over and over again. They obsess about one meal they think is unhealthy or that they regret eating. This leads them to justify additional treats ("Well, I already had one brownie, so the day is ruined; might as well have another") or unhealthy eating the rest of the week ("Well, I already had one bad meal, so the week is ruined"). A fender bender does not justify taking your car to the car crusher, so don't use one less-than-optimal meal as a reason to self-sabotage. Instead of obsessing about that meal, resolve to have a healthy meal or snack the next time you eat—and then do it.

Trying to be perfect with food does *not* work. Instead, to ensure lasting change, strategically balance your meals, snacks, and treats while remaining positive about your body and your health. Remember that we all eat, and food is not the enemy but rather a cultural celebration and the key to optimal health.

The Truth About Salt and High Blood Pressure

If you have high blood pressure, it's true that salt can make it worse. But salt does not necessarily *cause* high blood pressure if you don't have the condition already. It's also true that highly processed foods contain high amounts of sodium and sugar, making them hyper-palatable and addictive.

All that being said, salt-free is not necessarily healthier. When cooking at home, salt adds flavor and often brightens or dampens the taste of other ingredients. It can also be used to tenderize meat and draw water out of vegetables to allow them to roast properly. With my clients, I like to focus on increasing magnesium- and potassium-rich foods rather than cutting salt out of the diet. Magnesium and potassium combat the effects of sodium.

If you already have high blood pressure, it is important to be diligent about sodium. To control or prevent high blood pressure, focus on increasing plant-based foods in your diet.

IDENTIFY THE HABITS THAT STOP YOU FROM REACHING YOUR GOALS

"Bad" habits are usually a sign that you aren't practicing enough of a good habit. Instead of focusing on what you are doing wrong, focus on adding a healthy habit. On the left side of the chart on page 8 are common habits I've observed while working with clients over the years that make weight loss harder. On the right are healthy goals you can work on every month until you've mastered the healthy habit.

HABIT	HEALTHY GOAL
Eating too fast	Remove distractions at mealtime—no phone, TV, computer, or eating while driving. Put your fork down between bites.
Overeating Emotional eating Eating out of boredom	Ask yourself on a scale of 1 to 10 how hungry you are before you eat; then eat until you are no longer hungry (about 80 percent full).
Craving foods or often reaching for sugar	Eat enough protein at meals—at least 4 to 6 ounces, or 20 to 30 grams, of protein per meal. Eat at least 4 to 5 fistfuls of nonstarchy veggies per day. Drink half your body weight in fluid ounces of water every day. Sleep 8 hours minimum a night.
Snacking mindlessly	Record what you eat daily.
Drinking more than three cups of coffee a day or drinking sugar-sweetened beverages	Drink half your body weight in fluid ounces of water every day.
Feeling hungry soon after meals	Include a protein and a healthy fat in every meal.

SETTING GOALS

Benjamin Franklin once said, "If you fail to plan, you are planning to fail." Setting the right goals will give you a plan for success, while setting the wrong goals will set you up for failure. Most unhelpful are the ones that are vague, unrealistic, or unwanted and that lack a deadline.

There is also a *big* difference between setting short-term goals and long-term goals. Healthy weight loss takes time. The faster you lose weight, the more likely you are to gain it back. The slower the weight loss, the less your body will fight you every step of the way and the less likely you are to be a yo-yo dieter.

So how do you set a goal that can help you instead of hurting you? Your goals should be SMART—specific, measurable, achievable, realistic, and time-based. For your weight loss plan, about 1 pound a week is a healthy goal. To set a long-term SMART goal, determine how much weight you want to lose by a certain date—keeping in mind 1 pound a week. Then set short-term goals to help you get to your long-term goals. Your short-term goals can be how much weight you want to lose this month and how you will do it.

Let's say that you set a goal on January 1 to lose 50 pounds of body fat in one year based on the healthy goal of 1 pound of body fat lost per week. This is your long-term goal. Your short-term goal would be to lose 4 pounds of body fat by February 1 by eating four servings of veggies a day and drinking half your weight in fluid ounces of water every day. This goal is highly *specific*; it uses numbers and is therefore *measurable*; it is *achievable*, since it is based on things you are capable of doing; it is *realistic* based on facts about healthy weight loss; and it is *time-based*.

It's important to reward yourself for meeting your short-term goals with nonfood rewards, such as treating yourself to a massage, going to the movies, getting new clothes, buying a new book, or anything else relaxing and fulfilling that you love doing.

Also, keep in mind that weight loss doesn't have to be your ultimate goal. You may be more focused on health-related goals that include some weight loss as a means to get there. For example, do you want to get off or reduce medications for health conditions such as high blood pressure or high blood sugar? If so, that should be a long-term goal.

Understanding Calories and Portion Control

In this book, I'll teach you how to balance your meals so that you will feel full and avoid counting calories. The fewer processed foods you eat, the fewer cravings you will have and the fewer calories your body will naturally consume. However, I know that many of you prefer to count calories or feel you would learn from the experience. If this is you, I want to share some vital information about calories with you.

Your body has something called a basal metabolic rate, or BMR. It is the number of calories you need to operate the necessary processes to keep you alive, such as breathing and keeping your heart beating. Although everyone's BMR will vary due to age, gender, hormones, muscle mass, and other factors, your estimated BMR can be quickly calculated by multiplying your ideal body weight by 10.

Your ideal body weight is actually a range to fall within, not just one single number. I recommend the Hamwi method for a quick and easy calculation.

To calculate your ideal body weight using this method, begin with 100 pounds for females and 106 pounds for males. Now measure your height. Calculate how many inches you are above 5 feet. Multiply that number by 5 for females and by 6 for males. Finally, add that number to the base weight you started with—100 or 106 pounds. To find a range, calculate 10 percent above and below that final number.

For example, I'm female, so I'll begin with 100. I'm 5 feet 6 inches—6 inches taller than 5 feet—so I multiply 6 by 5 to make 30. Add that to 100 for a total of 130. Ten percent of 130 is 13, so my ideal body weight range is 117 to 143 pounds. Here is a quick summary, with this example written out in a few simple equations.

Calculating Ideal Body Weight Range

Males: 106 pounds + (6 pounds for each inch over 5 feet tall)

Females: 100 pounds + (5 pounds for each inch over 5 feet tall)

Your ideal body weight range is + or − 10 percent of this figure.

5-foot-6 female = 100 pounds + (5 × 6) = 130 pounds

130 × 10 percent = 13

+10 percent = 130 + 13 = 143

−10 percent = 130 − 13 = 117

Ideal body weight for a 5-foot-6 female is between 117 and 143 pounds.

Let's now do a quick basal metabolic rate calculation, continuing to use me, a 5-foot-6 female, as an example. First, calculate the BMR by multiplying your ideal body weight by 10. Use the middle of your weight range; for me, that would be 130. Multiply that by 10, and my BMR would be roughly 1,300. This is the number of calories required to keep me alive if I was not moving around, eating, or doing any nonessential activities.

I'm sure you know that you must burn more calories than you eat to lose weight, but a large deficit is not always better. In fact, it's rarely better for long-term weight loss. Let me explain.

When people take in fewer calories than their required BMR, their body understands this constant calorie deprivation as starvation and focuses only on staying alive. If I followed a strict diet of 1,200 calories per day, rather than my BMR of 1,300, my metabolism would go down so I could live on 1,200 calories, pushing my BMR to 1,200 or lower. If I continued to eat fewer calories per day, the cycle would continue.

It's also worth noting that the simple method of calculating BMR should not be used for daily calorie counting. Even though my ideal body weight is 130, when I've had my BMR tested, it's usually closer to 1,500. This is because I exercise and have built up my muscle mass; if I consistently ate fewer than 1,500 calories a day, I'd be harming my health.

If you genuinely want to count calories, I recommend using the steps in the box on page 12 to more accurately calculate both BMR and your total daily energy expenditure (TDEE), which is equal to your BMR, plus daily activity, plus digestion.

The number of calories you should consume for weight loss needs to be below your TDEE but above your BMR. Eating below your BMR requirements will cause you to have difficulty losing weight in the long term because it causes thyroid and sex hormone disruptions that upset your natural metabolism.

Calculating Basal Metabolic Rate (BMR) and Total Daily Energy Expenditure

Begin by converting your weight from pounds to kilograms and your height from inches to centimeters. You will use these numbers to calculate your BMR.

1. Convert weight in pounds to kilograms: _____ pounds ÷ 2.2 = _____ kilograms

2. Convert height in inches to centimeters: _____ inches × 2.54 = _____ centimeters

3. Calculate basal metabolic rate (BMR) using the Harris-Benedict equation:

Male BMR = 66.5 + (13.75 × weight in kilograms) + (5.003 × height in centimeters) − (age × 6.775)

Female BMR = 655.1 + (9.563 × weight in kilograms) + (1.850 × height in centimeters) − (age × 4.676)

Let's use me as an example again, a 130-pound, 5-foot-6, 35-year-old female.

130 pounds ÷ 2.2 = 59.1 kilograms

I am 5 foot 6. That's 66 inches (5 × 12 = 60 + 6 = 66).

66 inches × 2.54 = 167.64 centimeters

Here's what the calculation for my BMR would look like:

655.1 + (9.563 × 59.1) + (1.850 × 167.64) − (35 × 4.676) = 1,366.74

Now, to calculate TDEE, consider your activity level, and choose an activity factor number from the following chart.

ACTIVITY LEVEL	ACTIVITY FACTOR
Sedentary (little or no exercise)	1.2
Lightly active (exercise 1 to 3 days a week)	1.375
Moderately active (exercise 3 to 5 days a week)	1.55
Very active (exercise 6 or 7 days a week)	1.725
Extremely active (vigorous exercise 2 or more times a day)	1.9

To find your TDEE, take the BMR rate you just calculated and multiply it by your activity factor. The equation looks like this:

BMR × activity factor = TDEE

Let's use me as an example one more time. My BMR is 1,366.74. Let's say I'm lightly active; that means my activity factor is 1.375.

1,366.74 × 1.375 = 1,879.27

So my TDEE is 1,879.27. This means that to maintain an ideal weight of 130 pounds with consistent light activity, I need to eat more than 1,367 calories (my BMR) but less than 1,879 calories per day.

Note: The low end of this range is still significantly less than the 1,500 calories I mentioned earlier. This is why I use body fat percentage to calculate macro and calorie needs for myself and my clients. If you have been working out consistently for a long time, consider having your macros calculated by a qualified professional who uses body fat percentage. For most people, though, this won't be necessary.

ALL CALORIES ARE NOT CREATED EQUAL

While you must be in a calorie deficit to lose weight, it's essential to understand that not all calories are created equal. Fifteen hundred calories of processed foods such as French fries, candy, and chips are not the same as 1,500 calories of whole foods such as veggies, lean meats, whole grains, and healthy fats.

Your body has to do extra work to digest and eliminate the preservatives, chemicals, sugar, salt, and refined carbohydrates in processed foods. Furthermore, processed foods lack the nutrients such as vitamins, minerals, antioxidants, and phytochemicals that you need in addition to protein, fats, and fiber for optimal health. When your body is missing these essential nutrients, it will continue to crave food, even if your calorie needs have been met. And while these foods will give you a quick energy boost, you will experience a crash later on, causing you to crave more foods with added sugar and refined carbohydrates.

To get off the merry-go-round, choose nutrient-dense, whole, real foods as much as possible rather than processed foods.

Optimizing Your Pantry

I find that the majority of my clients are not eating too much. Instead, they're not eating enough of the right foods, which include as much produce as possible, followed by whole grains, lean meats, and healthy fats.

FOODS TO RESTRICT

When you're eating a healthy diet, choose whole foods over processed, refined foods, which lack nutrients and just function as empty calories. Here is a list of foods I avoid in my own home:

Bleached and unbleached flours and grains: These include all-purpose white flour, gluten-free one-to-one blends, and white rice.

Refined sugars: These include cane sugar, fruit juice, and other processed sweeteners.

Unfamiliar ingredients: That means any food with more than two ingredients on the label that you don't recognize as food. Foods with more than five ingredients total are also suspect.

Foods with dyes, chemicals, or preservatives

Sugar-sweetened beverages: These include sports drinks, coffee drinks, sweetened teas, energy drinks, juice (including 100 percent fruit juice), soda, and other sweetened drinks.

Artificial sweeteners: These trick your brain into thinking you're having sugar and rewire your taste buds to expect unnaturally sweet food.

FOODS TO ENJOY IN MODERATION

These foods shouldn't be banned from your home, but you should consume them in moderation. *Moderation* is a word that means something different to every person, so just keep track of these foods to be sure you don't overdo it.

Natural low-calorie sweeteners: These include stevia, monk fruit, chicory, and xylitol. These are good alternatives to artificial sweeteners because they are low-calorie, but they are still much sweeter than most foods. Limit their use to once a day.

Natural sweeteners: These include maple syrup, coconut sugar, honey, raw cane sugar, and agave syrup. They have the same amount of sugar as a teaspoon of refined sugar but also contain trace minerals and, in general, may be better for blood sugar control.

Coffee: Stick to a maximum of two or three cups a day and enjoy it black or with cream and limited real sugar or natural sweeteners.

Tea: Stick to a maximum of two or three cups a day for all caffeinated beverages and enjoy it plain or with cream and a little real sugar or natural sweeteners. There's no limit to how much decaf and herbal tea you can drink.

Whole fruit: Enjoy fruit in all forms, including fresh, frozen, and canned. For weight loss, one or two servings of fruit a day is plenty.

Processed dairy and dairy alternatives: I'm equal opportunity when it comes to dairy and nondairy. Low-fat dairy is still the standard recommendation for a healthy diet, but there is generous research to support full-fat dairy for optimal health. If you would like to eat dairy, I recommend organic whole-fat dairy products to my clients because they're more filling. The more significant issue is that if you do consume dairy, you should avoid the added chemicals and sugar found in some dairy products. Dairy alternatives can be a good option for those who want or need to avoid dairy products. However, again, watch out for additives and preservatives.

Processed meats: Choose processed meats with care and limit how much you eat in a week to two servings. Choose uncured, nitrate-free processed meats such as bacon, lunch meat, and sausages. There is a strong association between processed meats and colon cancer. However, these associations do not equal causation and do not account for nitrate-free varieties.

FOODS TO ENJOY LIBERALLY

The Produce for Better Health Foundation, a nonprofit organization commit-ted to helping people learn to enjoy eating fruits and vegetables, recommends that you remember the simple message to "Have a Plant" with each of your meals. This message is simple but effective for better health and faster weight loss. The more plants you have every day, the better! Always strive to pick food in its least processed form.

Nonstarchy vegetables: Anything other than peas, corn, potatoes, sweet potatoes, and winter squash counts as a nonstarchy veggie and can be eaten liberally. All types are healthy, including fresh, frozen, and canned. Always have nonstarchy vegetables on hand.

Starchy vegetables: These include peas, corn, potatoes, sweet pota-toes, and winter squash, all of which are good sources of fiber-rich carbohydrates.

A variety of whole grains: These include brown rice, oats, quinoa, whole wheat, and other grains. They can come in the form of the grain itself, such as brown rice, or bread, pasta, and other products—as long as they're whole-grain.

Beans and lentils: These are fiber-rich and great pantry staples in all forms, including dry and canned. Canned beans are convenient, last a long time, and can easily be rinsed to remove excess salt.

Nuts and seeds: These are filling, great for hormone balance, and a staple in a healthy diet. Each type of nut or seed has its own unique nutrition benefits, and no one specific choice is better than the other, so include a variety for optimal health.

Seafood: Try to eat seafood at least twice a week, since it provides lean protein and essential omega-3 fatty acids that fight inflammation. Wild-caught seafood is always a good choice, but some sustainably farmed fish options are healthy as well. When in doubt, follow the Monte-rey Bay Aquarium's Seafood Watch list (seafoodwatch.org) when buying seafood. The concern with eating too much seafood is mercury contam-ination. The biggest fish that are highest on the food chain tend to have the most mercury; these include (but are not limited to) swordfish, shark, mackerel, and albacore tuna. Limit consuming these to twice a week to avoid mercury overload; other types of fish you can eat without limits. For where you can find a full list of seafood and mercury levels broken into low, medium, and high, see Resources (page 195).

Poultry: Chicken and turkey are naturally leaner than other forms of protein and provide many essential nutrients.

Eggs: Eggs are a source of 11 essential nutrients. Though they were once vilified for their cholesterol, research shows that dietary cholesterol intake does not influence cholesterol levels in most healthy people. Unless you have a genetic predisposition to absorbing cholesterol at a higher rate, you should enjoy eggs liberally on a healthy diet.

100 percent grass-fed meat: I am incredibly passionate about 100 percent grass-fed meat. It's better for the planet and your body because it contains more antioxidants and more omega-3s and is naturally leaner. If you can't afford it, buy very lean meat because toxins are stored in the fat of animals.

Pork: Pork can be part of a healthy diet and supplies many nutrients, but choose leaner cuts.

Unprocessed dairy: As I mentioned earlier, heavily processed dairy with added sugars, preservatives, and chemicals should be consumed in moderation. However, unprocessed organic dairy, such as plain full-fat milk, yogurt, cottage cheese, and cheese, can be consumed liberally.

Healthy cooking oils: Consider these pantry staples. Some of my favorites are extra-virgin olive oil, avocado oil, coconut oil, and sesame oil.

All kinds of vinegar and natural condiments: Feel free to include vinegars and condiments in a healthy diet. Just read the ingredients list to make sure there are no preservatives and fillers. Five ingredients or less is great, unless you notice that all the ingredients are recognizable as real food.

30 Days to Transformation

Over the next 30 days, you will have moments of success and moments of stagnation or less noticeable progress. You may try a recipe you don't like or not see the scale move in the way you expected and think you failed. These are the times you may want to give up, but it's moving past these challenges and understanding them as learning experiences that will make you successful. Success comes only after pushing past the harder moments.

MINOR OBSTACLES

Each obstacle is just a challenge; you will see the fruits of your labor only if you push past the obstacles. You will not be able to control every meal, you will not always say no to the office junk food, you will not always work out when scheduled, the scale will not always show weight loss, and you will not love every recipe in this book. You will not always want to eat healthy. Do it anyway. And when you fall off the track, get back on. If you eat unhealthy, eat healthy for the next meal. If you miss a workout, work out the next day. Don't let a minor obstacle or setback turn into another year of excuses. As the Nike ads say, just do it.

MAJOR AWESOMENESS

And if you do it, what will be your reward? Major awesomeness. I'm not kidding. Yes, you will eventually see that scale move, you will have fewer cravings for sugar, you'll be able to enjoy one cookie instead of ten, you will find healthy recipes you love, and you will find it easier and easier to stay on track. As you eat healthier, you will provide your body with nutrients that will fight chronic disease, help you lose weight, increase your energy, and make you feel 10 years younger. It's not a pill, it's a lifestyle. It starts with you—right now.

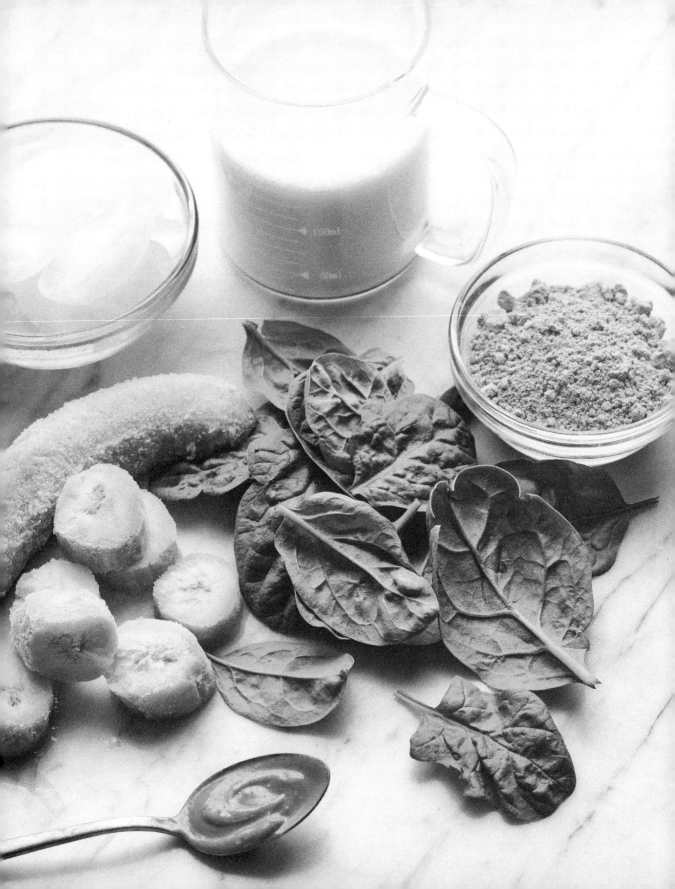

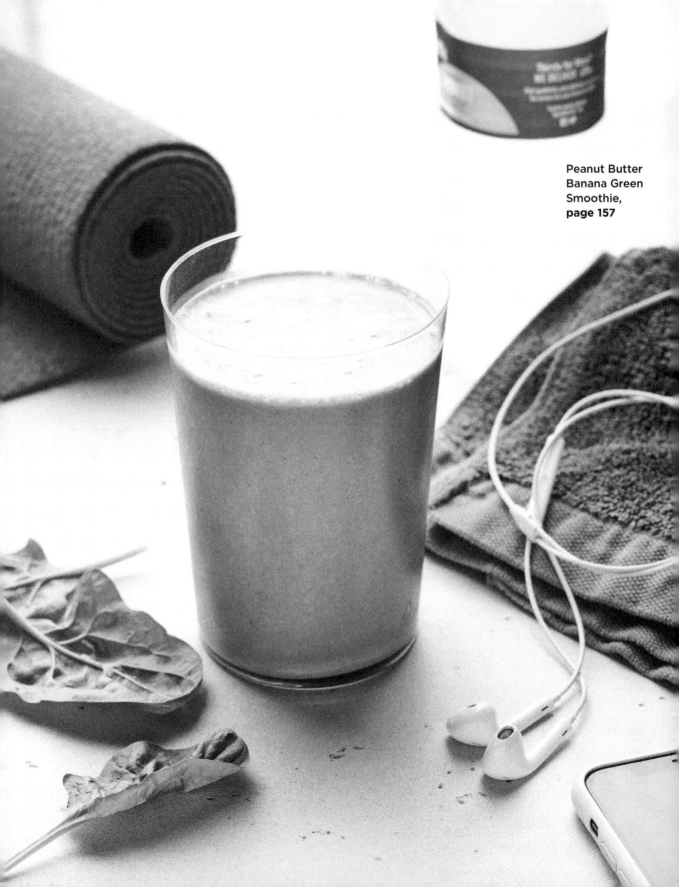

Peanut Butter
Banana Green
Smoothie,
page 157

CHAPTER 2

Exercise

EXERCISE NOT ONLY HELPS YOU LOSE WEIGHT BY BURNING calories but also helps your body function optimally at the cellular level. It improves how your body uses calories, reduces the risk of heart disease, enhances cognition, and improves your mood. It quite literally changes your body inside and out to perform at its best, feel its best, and function at its best. In this chapter, I'll review best practices for exercise and provide recommendations for your 30-day plan and beyond.

Set an Exercise Routine

The trainers you see bouncing around with rock-hard abs screaming about how great exercise is are not normal. What *is* normal is to initially hate exercise. Yes, I said it! It's not just you. Our bodies are designed to conserve energy for when we need it the most. We are hardwired to seek pleasure and avoid pain, and that's why we survive as a species. We seek pleasure in food, company, and rest. We avoid pain and use resources efficiently.

Think of it this way: People used to have to always be ready to hunt for food and defend their homes. So why would they waste energy going for a leisurely jog? It would exhaust them, and they wouldn't be ready to spring into action. Modern-day society isn't like that, though. We don't often find ourselves running from tigers and bears unless there's a mass escape at the local zoo.

Without basic survival on the line, you must find your own motivation to exercise, and that's not always easy. However, it's extremely necessary; the human body was built to move, proven by the fact that the benefits of exercise are unending. Just a little bit of exercise a day—between 30 minutes and an hour (depending on the type of exercise)—protects your health and changes your bodily functions, both inside and out, down to the cellular level.

So, if exercise doesn't feel natural, how do you get it done? You first have to make time for it in your day. At the beginning of each week, schedule your workouts like appointments. Think of them as the most important appointment in your day, one you cannot miss. As a personal trainer, I've found that people who prioritize exercise at the beginning of their day are more successful than those who wait until the evening to work out. The morning exercisers are more consistent, lose more weight, and stay the course. Of course, I've had clients do well exercising in the evening too, but as an overall observation, the early birds more often get the worm.

You'll have to figure out what works for you, and that may take some trial and error. It will take a few months to build the habit of exercise, and it will take even longer, maybe even a few years, before you become one of those people who can't live without exercise. Eventually, though, you'll find the type of training that motivates you and excites you.

When you're starting to explore different types of exercise, you may want to know what will give you the most bang for your buck or which kind of training you should do and how often. To start, let's break down the different types of exercise.

CARDIOVASCULAR EXERCISE

Cardiovascular exercise is anything that raises your heart rate and breathing, thereby training your cardiovascular system to expand its capacity. The most traditional cardio is sustained moderate-intensity aerobic exercise, such as running, spinning (riding a stationary bike), stair climbing, and swimming, though any exercise that raises your heart rate counts.

It's important to include cardio in your weekly routine because it expands your ability to take in oxygen and improves the efficiency with which your heart pumps blood. The goal is to increase your heart's and body's capacity to withstand stress.

For example, if you're a beginner, running up one flight of stairs might make you winded. After training your cardiovascular system (with or without weight loss), you will be able to run up one flight of stairs without breaking a sweat.

The biggest mistake I see people making over and over again is including only one type of cardio in their weekly fitness routine. It's important to include all three of the following:

Low-intensity steady state (LISS) cardio includes longer periods of low-intensity workouts. For example, if you take a 45- to 60-minute brisk walk or light jog, your heart rate is up, but you aren't gasping for air the whole time, and you could easily maintain a light conversation.

Moderate-intensity cardio means you are pushing yourself, but you are not out of breath. It's the sweet spot where you can't quite hold a conversation but feel you could keep up the intensity for at least 30 minutes. A good example of this level of cardio is running for 30 minutes at a pace that makes you feel comfortable, though you could not maintain a conversation.

High-intensity interval training (HIIT) brings you to the brink of your anaerobic threshold, or your ability to function with limited oxygen. Interval training means short periods (20 to 90 seconds) of high-level work with longer periods of low- or moderate-intensity work in between. The workout time is limited to about 20 minutes.

Many people make the mistake of doing only long cardio sessions or becoming obsessed with the endorphin rush of HIIT workouts while disregarding the other types of cardio. For the most effective training, all three should be in your weekly routine.

STRENGTH TRAINING

Strength training is of equal importance to cardiovascular exercise. Read that again: I said *equal*, and I meant it, friend.

I find that when people are trying to lose weight, they throw strength training to the side in favor of long cardio sessions that burn calories. This is a mistake. The muscle mass we carry is more metabolically active than fat—a whole lot more. As we age, we lose our muscle mass slowly, unless we halt some of that loss. When you're trying to lose weight, this becomes *very* important.

If you don't include strength training in your weight loss exercise program, your body will start to break down muscle tissue instead of fat. But when you lose weight, you want to lose fat, not muscle. Losing muscle slows down your metabolism and requires you to work harder to maintain your weight loss.

Strength training uses your body weight and/or weight-training tools to provide resistance to the body, with the goal of increasing the size, strength, and endurance of muscle fibers. It can prevent muscle loss while you are losing weight and even help you gain strength.

Furthermore, a strength workout may not burn as many calories as a cardio session initially, but it burns them for a lot longer. Including strength training in your workouts means you'll burn more calories for 12 to 24 hours after the workout has ended, versus cardio where the calorie burn ends when the workout ends. This is known as the exercise post-oxygen consumption (EPOC) effect, and it's elevated as your body tries to repair and recover muscle mass.

The three-day exercise plan in this chapter will recommend both cardio and strength training throughout the week so that you obtain all the benefits from all types of exercise and get the best results.

STRETCHING AND FOAM ROLLING

Stretching is an essential part of your exercise program because over-tight muscles can lead to injuries and pain. Stretching after a workout lengthens muscle fibers and helps you safely cool down post-workout.

Many people also find foam rolling tight muscle groups to be beneficial. A foam roller is a cheap tube made out of fairly hard foam that you can place on the floor and roll over muscle groups, like a self-massage, to help tight muscles relax and reduce post-exercise soreness.

This plan will not include specific stretching recommendations because every single person's body is different and what might feel good to one person could lead to injury in another. I recommend foam rolling at least once a week and stretching either as part of your active recovery on your rest days (the days you don't work out but do something to keep moving), as in yoga, or at the end of your workout. Some helpful stretches include targeting large muscle groups such as the following:

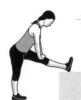

→ **Hamstrings:** Stand up straight with your feet slightly apart. Place your right ankle on the edge of a block or a chair in front of you that is at knee-height. Placing your hands at the top of your thigh, lean forward as much as you can without feeling pain. Release and do the other side. You should feel the stretch in the back of the top part of your leg where the hamstring muscles are located.

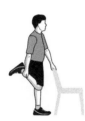

→ **Quadriceps:** Standing on one leg, bend the other leg behind you, grasp the ankle, and pull that leg back to your buttocks. Make sure your knees stay in line. You should feel the stretch in the front of the top part of your leg where your quadriceps are located.

→ **Inner thigh muscles:** Sit in a butterfly position with your knees bent and the soles of your feet touching each other. Bend forward slightly until you feel a stretch in your inner thighs.

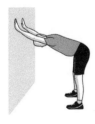

→ **Midback:** These stretches are great for your back. Holding on to a wall or bar, move your hips backward as your arms extend over your head, until your body forms an inverted *L* with your face looking down at the floor. You should feel the stretch in the middle of your back, where the latissimus dorsi muscles, known as lats, are located.

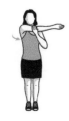

→ **Shoulders:** One arm at a time, bring your arm across your chest. You should feel the stretch in the middle of your back behind your shoulder blades.

Selecting Weights

It's important that you learn to select the right weights for your body. Keep a set of light, medium, and heavy weights for different exercises. How do you select the right weights? You should be able to maintain good form for every rep of the exercise. For higher rep counts (15 to 20 per exercise), you will need to be able to hold the correct form the entire time, so you will need lighter weights than for a lower-rep scheme (5 to 10 per exercise) because you have more reps to do. If you can no longer maintain your form with a selected weight but still have reps left, lower the weight and continue your reps. Similar rules apply to time-based exercises. Typically, in a time-based exercise, you should be shooting to complete 12 to 15 reps in 1 minute. If you can do more than that, increase the weight. If you can't quite reach that, decrease the weight.

Time-based weight exercises:

30 seconds: 5 to 8 reps

45 seconds: 8 to 12 reps

60 seconds: 12 to 15 reps

90 seconds: 15 to 20 reps

For bodyweight exercises, move as quickly as possible while maintaining good form.

Go-To Exercise Circuits

These are my go-to exercise circuits. They are effective and don't waste any time! Each circuit takes about 30 minutes to complete. I recommend using a Tabata timer app on your phone to keep track of the time in these exercises. (There are plenty of free ones available.)

STRENGTH AND CARDIO CIRCUIT

This strength and cardio combination circuit is intended to keep your heart rate up and burn calories while also building strength. Incorporating strength into a cardio routine also boosts the EPOC effect, which is how many calories you'll burn after the workout.

Start with a two-round warm-up; do each exercise for 1 minute, and then repeat the whole sequence.

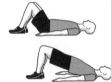

1. **1-minute glute bridges:** Lie on your back with your feet planted on the ground, raise your hips toward the ceiling, and then lower them back down. That's 1 rep. Repeat for 1 minute.

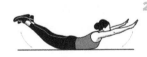

2. **1-minute Supermans:** Lie on your stomach, raise both your arms and both your legs off the floor at the same time, pause at the top, and then come back down. That's 1 rep. Repeat for 1 minute.

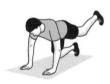

3. **1-minute donkey kicks:** Get on all fours and kick one leg back while slightly raising it. Your leg should be fully extended and you should feel it in your glute muscle. Raise and lower your leg for 30 seconds on each side.

Then complete three rounds of the entire circuit. In each round, repeat each exercise for 1 minute, and then move on to the next exercise.

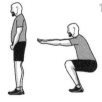

1. **Air squats:** Stand up straight with your feet slightly apart; then lower your body down as if you were sitting on an invisible chair behind you. At the bottom of the squat, your quads should be parallel to the floor, your feet should be flat on the floor, and your knees should

be over your toes but not extending past them. Your arms should be straight out in front of you and parallel to the floor. To make this exercise harder, hold a weight (dumbbell, kettlebell, 1-gallon water bottle, whatever you have) at your chest.

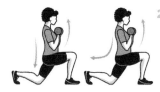

2. **Reverse lunges:** Stand up straight with your feet slightly apart. Step back with the right leg and lower both legs until they are both bent 90 degrees but don't touch the floor. Then come back up and step your right leg back to center. Complete this on both the left and right sides, 30 seconds per side.

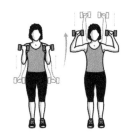

3. **Biceps curl to Arnold press:** Stand up straight with your feet slightly apart. Hold a dumbbell in each hand with your palms facing away from your body and your arms straight down by your side. Now bend your elbows and curl your arms in toward your body to bring your arms up to your shoulders. Next, extend your arms up until they are straight over your head. As you lift the weights, turn your palms so they face out, away from your body. Reverse the motion to come back down.

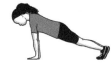

4. **Push-ups:** Position your body in a plank pose (the top of a push-up with your arms extended, supporting your body), with your hands under your shoulders and a flat back. Do not let your back or your rear end drop down. (You can lower your knees to the floor for a modified push-up.) Slowly lower yourself down until your chest almost touches the ground; then raise yourself back up.

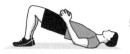

5. **Glute bridges (with a weight):** This move is identical to the glute bridges in the warm-ups, but hold a weight on your hips while performing the movement.

6. **Cardio:** Finally, spend 5 minutes on an elliptical machine or any cardio machine, switching between 30 seconds of work (going as hard as you can) and 30 seconds of recovery (still moving but taking it easy). If you don't have a machine, jumping rope is a great alternative.

Repeat the entire circuit, including the cardio, twice more.

FULL-BODY CIRCUIT

This circuit is designed to work small stabilizing muscles as well as big muscle groups for an allover full-body workout. It is split into four mini circuits that take about 9 minutes each. Within each circuit, complete three rounds of each exercise, with each round taking about 1 minute.

MINI CIRCUIT 1

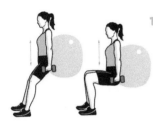

1. **Sumo squat:** Stand with your feet slightly wider than shoulder-width apart. Begin to squat; as you lower down, your knees will turn outward over your toes. In this squat, you want to lower down until your thighs are lower than parallel with the floor—or as low as you can get while your feet remain flat on the floor and your knees do not extend past your toes. For added challenge, place an exercise ball against a wall and perform the squat while maintaining a light, constant pressure against the ball. Repeat for 1 minute.

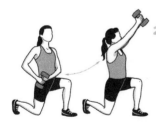

2. **Half-kneeling wood chops:** Start by kneeling on the floor. Lift your left foot and place it in front of you on the floor so your left knee is bent 90 degrees and you're now kneeling on just your right knee. Use both hands to hold a weight next to your right hip. With control and keeping your arms straight, raise the weight above your head in one motion. Bring it back down to the starting position. Continue this motion for 1 minute on the left and 1 minute on the right side for each round. Repeat twice more on each side for a total of 3 minutes per side.

MINI CIRCUIT 2

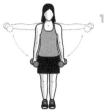

1. **Lateral raises:** Stand with your feet shoulder-width apart. With your arms at your sides, hold a dumbbell in each hand with your palms facing your body. Raise both arms straight up to either side, until they form a *T* and your palms are facing down. With control, bring them back down. Repeat for 1 minute.

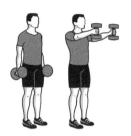

2. **Front raises:** Stand with your feet shoulder-width apart. With your arms at your sides, hold a dumbbell in each hand with your palms facing your body. Raise both arms in front of you until they're shoulder height. Your palms should be facing each other but the dumbbells should not be touching. With control, bring them back down to the starting position. Repeat for 1 minute.

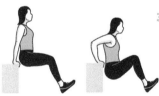

3. **Bench or chair dips:** Stand with the backs of your legs touching the seat of a sturdy chair or the edge of a bench. Lower yourself until you can place your palms flat on the chair or bench with your fingers pointed toward yourself. With your legs straight out in front of you (or bent, for an easier variation), keep your back close to the chair or bench while you bend your elbows to lower yourself down, and then press back up with your arms. Repeat for 1 minute.

MINI CIRCUIT 3

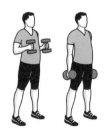

1. **Hammer curls:** Stand up straight with your feet slightly apart. Hold a dumbbell in each hand with your palms facing each other. Bend your arms so the weights come up to your shoulders; keep your palms facing each other but not touching. With control, lower the weights back down. Repeat for 1 minute.

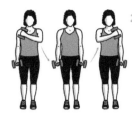

2. **Cross-body curls:** Stand up straight with your feet slightly apart. Hold a dumbbell in each hand with your palms facing out away from the body. Lift one weight to tap the opposite shoulder; your palms should face outward and then turn to face the shoulder. With control, bring the weights back down. Repeat on the other side. Repeat the whole exercise for 1 minute.

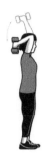

3. **Overhead triceps extensions:** Stand up straight with your feet slightly apart. Hold a dumbbell in each hand with your palms facing each other. Extend your arms straight up above your head like goal posts. Bend your elbows 90 degrees to lower the weights behind the back of your head. With control, bring the weights back up. Repeat for 1 minute.

MINI CIRCUIT 4

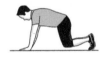

1. **Bear plank:** Get on all fours; then lift your knees so they hover 2 inches above the floor. Keep your back flat. Hold for 3 to 5 seconds, and then lower. Repeat for 1 minute.

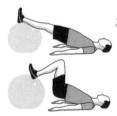

2. **Hamstring sliders:** Lie on your back with your knees bent and your feet flat on the floor. Place a slider exercise mat, an exercise ball or a towel underneath your feet. Lift your hips slightly and extend your legs until they are straight, or as far as you can without letting your buttocks touch the floor. Then bring them back to the starting position. Repeat for 1 minute.

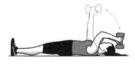

3. **Skull crushers:** Lie on your back. Hold a dumbbell in each hand with your palms facing each other and your arms extended straight up. Bend your elbows as you lower the weights down to your head. With control, bring the weights back up. Repeat for 1 minute.

CARDIO HIIT CIRCUIT

This HIIT circuit is as fast as it is efficient. It takes 30 minutes to get head-to-toe drenched in sweat! Start with a 5-minute warm-up, and then spend 20 minutes on any cardio machine—or go for a bike ride, run, or brisk walk. Whatever method you choose, switch between 60 seconds of work and 60 seconds of recovery. After 20 minutes, complete a 5-minute cooldown (such as a light jog or walk) to wrap up your workout.

Warm-ups and cooldowns can be anything that gets your body moving. The idea is to not jump into or out of vigorous exercise too quickly. Some great ideas are walking, light jogging, or doing some other easy exercise.

Exercise Myths

Let's bust some common exercise myths. These are the ones I hear most often from my clients and blog readers:

1. **"Cardio is the best for weight loss."** While cardio is important, a mix of cardio and strength training is the best way to lose weight, increase fitness, and achieve lasting results.

2. **"Strength training will make you bulky."** This is a complaint mostly from women, but rest assured, it's tough to get bulky, especially while losing weight. First of all, to put on a ton of muscle mass, you need a ton of testosterone—a hormone that females don't produce much of. Second, you'd have to be in a sustained calorie surplus. For body-builders to put on mass, they must intentionally gain weight and put themselves in a calorie surplus. So unless you are lifting maximum weight, eating way more than you need, and producing a boatload of testosterone, you won't get bulky. You might get sleek lines, though, making you look toned and fit.

3. **"You can lose fat in just one area."** It's impossible to spot-reduce some areas of your body while preserving other areas. When you lose weight, you must lose it all over, and you have no control over where it comes off first or last. That being said, you can work the muscle group in a specific area so that as you lose weight, the muscles underneath pop and look toned earlier.

4. **"You need to stretch before you work out."** Research has shown that traditional stretching may reduce power and maybe even increase injury when working out, but the jury is still out on that one. Instead, it would be best if you focused on a dynamic warm-up, in which you stretch and move lightly for no more than 3 to 5 seconds in each stretch, saving the long, static stretching for after your workout.

Getting the Most Out of Your Workouts

Now that we've busted some exercise myths, here's how to get the most out of your workout:

1. **Incorporate strength training and cardio.**

2. **Vary the intensity level.** Not every workout should be balls to the wall. That's a sure way to stress your hormones and burn yourself out fast. Additionally, not every workout should be a leisurely jog where you barely break a sweat, since you won't make progress. Include a variety of intensity levels and types of workouts throughout the week to get the best results.

3. **Track your progress.** Keep a journal of your workouts and track data points, including which weights you use and how long the workout takes, so you can see your progress.

4. **Follow a progressive program.** This is a program in which you track your progress and keep changing things up, moving through different rep and time schemes to continually challenge yourself.

5. **Drink plenty of water.** Drink half your body weight in fluid ounces of water every day for maximal recovery. In other words, if you weigh 130 pounds, drink 65 ounces of water every day.

6. **Choose protein and carbs after a workout.** For maximal recovery, eat a protein and a carbohydrate after your workout. My favorite is a premade protein shake with an added banana; it's easy, portable, and delicious.

Recommendations

In your 30-day plan, I include recommendations for weekly workouts—switching between cardio and strength training—to help you get started. However, it will be up to you to find a type of exercise that you enjoy. When you're looking for new workout programs to try, use the following guidelines to decide whether to begin the program as is or modify it:

1. **Include at least one rest day a week.** Most people need at least one or two rest days per week. These rest days can include active recovery such as stretching, gentle yoga, foam rolling, or leisurely walks or bike rides. However, rest days shouldn't include anything that gets your heart rate up or interferes with recovery from your other workouts during the week. Skipping rest days will stress your body out and you won't see results—or worse, you'll get injured.

2. **Do strength and resistance training.** It's best to include strength training at least two and preferably three times a week. For beginners, I recommend full-body circuits instead of training only one muscle group at a time. While "leg" day and "arm" day can be great to make progress if you are already in great shape, beginners should focus on full-body workouts each time they train with weights. If you hit only one muscle group per week, you may not be able to work hard enough to make progress. In contrast, full-body training two or three times a week will enhance endurance and strength and lead to faster results.

3. **Vary the cardio intensity.** As previously discussed, you should vary the intensity of your cardio workouts throughout the week. Include one low-intensity steady state (LISS) workout per week (see page 23). Moderate-intensity and HIIT cardio may come in the form of strength training or traditional cardio activity. Be sure to have a solid mix of both of them because too much HIIT can stress your body out, while not enough HIIT can halt progress. Moderate intensity is the sweet spot and is often achieved with full-body strength training circuits, so it's a double bang for your buck!

To get you started, here's my recommended ideal workout schedule for one week. This list refers to the exercise circuits I've laid out in this chapter. But feel free to try different exercises and routines as you get more comfortable.

→ 1 cardio HIIT circuit

→ 1 strength and cardio circuit

→ 1 LISS workout

→ 2 full-body circuits

→ 2 active recovery or rest days

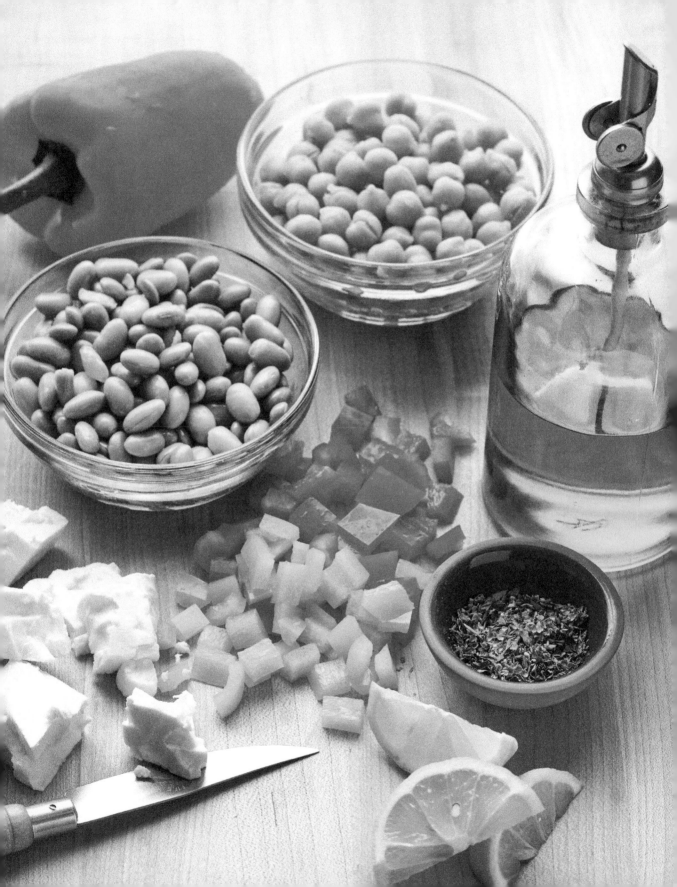

CHAPTER 3

Five Steps to Success

IN THIS CHAPTER WE WILL DISCUSS THE FIVE STEPS TO successful weight loss using this 30-day plan and other practices beyond this program. You will learn the most effective strategies for using this plan; how to prepare your kitchen and pantry; how to prepare the recipes; the best way to be more mindful when you eat; and the importance of sleep, relaxation, and exercise to your success. Let's jump in!

Plan Ahead

It's super important to use the meal plan to your full advantage by making it work for your life. So let's start by talking about creating and implementing a strategy for making this meal plan work for you. Of course, I've given you a weekly meal plan, but it has plenty of flexibility.

HOW TO USE THE MEAL PLAN

At first glance, I sincerely hope the meal plan looks doable. That's what I was going for when I designed it. However, you also have to think about the meal plan in terms of your life. Developing the habit of cooking almost every night is a big deal and could be a significant change from the way you eat now. That's okay! Look at the plan with a little flexibility and consider options such as meal prepping in advance or choosing the simpler recipes on your busiest days.

Just as you've scheduled your workouts for the week, consider planning your meals. Are there days when you know you'll be home late because you're shuttling the kids to and fro or you have a late shift at work? Make sure you plan the quickest meals for those days. Additionally, look at the days where you'll be home earlier and prepare the meals that take a little longer on those days.

You might be thinking, "I bought this book so that the work would already be done for me. Can't I just follow the meal plan without thinking about it?" Yes, you can! This meal plan is designed to be as simple as possible. Still, I think you'll find life a lot easier, and be more likely to stick with this 30-day plan, if you spent a few minutes rearranging things (if necessary) to fit your schedule. You'll still eat the same breakfast, lunch, snacks, and dinner mapped out in this book. It's just that you might find it easier to follow the Tuesday schedule on a Thursday or the Thursday schedule on a Monday, for example.

You'll notice that the meal plan includes leftovers, so you aren't cooking for every single meal. You will have to pay attention to where the leftovers fall, but this could work to your advantage. Again, if you can plan to use the leftovers on a day that you will be busier, go for it.

If your week looks jam-packed, you may want to consider prepping either entire meals or parts of meals in advance. If Wednesday looks impossibly busy, maybe you make both Tuesday and Wednesday dinners on Tuesday. Or if the entire week looks busy, doing small things like chopping up veggies or pre-cooking grains at the beginning of the week can make meals come together faster during the week.

Prepare Your Kitchen and Pantry

It's time to prep your kitchen and pantry. You might be thinking you need to throw out all the junk food in your house or you will never be successful. While this is an excellent time to clean out and evaluate your pantry, focus first on making sure you have what you need to make the meals in your meal plan. You can tackle the purge later.

USEFUL KITCHEN EQUIPMENT

I am assuming you have some kitchen basics: measuring cups and spoons, a medium saucepan with a lid, and aluminum foil. Consider making sure you also have these items before you get started:

Heavy-duty baking sheets: I love sheet pan recipes, but a cheap baking sheet can buckle at high heat, sending your food flying all over your oven. Make sure you have at least one or two heavy-duty baking sheets.

Blender: You can't make smoothies without one!

Large nonstick skillet: A good-quality nonstick skillet with a lid will make your life much easier.

Cooking oil mister/sprayer: Instead of cooking with unhealthy nonstick cooking sprays or overpaying for healthy ones, buy a refillable cooking oil sprayer.

Silicone spatulas of various sizes: I love silicone spatulas for all my cooking and baking because they work well to scrape out every last drop of batter. They also won't scratch nonstick cookware, which is important because nonstick cookware should be thrown out when it is damaged to avoid possible chemical contamination.

Chef's knife: When you are cooking at home every night, a good knife can make all the difference. A chef's knife has an 8- to 12-inch-long blade and is broad and sharp. It doesn't have to be expensive; just make sure your knife is sharp enough to facilitate quick chopping.

Cutting boards: My favorite cutting boards are plastic of different colors so it's easy to make sure I use different ones for meats and vegetables. They make it so easy to keep food safely separated, and they are dishwasher-safe.

HEALTHY PANTRY ESSENTIALS

Avocado oil and extra-virgin olive oil: Avocado oil has healthy fats similar to those in olive oil but with a much milder flavor and higher smoke point (for cooking at higher temperatures). Reserve the extra-virgin olive oil for cooking at very low temperatures and for cold food, such as salad dressings. The unrefined cold-pressed versions do not hold up to heat well; the versions that do hold up to heat are very heavily processed.

Rolled oats: Oats are so versatile! They're great to bake with, grind into flour, or use for a quick breakfast.

Canned tomatoes: You can use these in everything! I keep canned diced tomatoes in my pantry at all times. These are what I use most often because after you rinse them you can barely tell they are canned.

Dried seasonings: Salt, pepper, garlic, onion, and paprika are the seasonings I use most frequently, but I also love to use blends such as Italian seasoning, pizza seasoning, barbecue seasoning, taco seasoning, and Old Bay. Seasoning blends make it easy to quickly add flavor to any meal.

Whole grains: Your pantry should include a variety of whole grains such as brown rice, quinoa, and whole-grain pasta.

Step Three: **Prepare the Recipes**

If you're not used to cooking very often, this 30-day plan won't be easy—but it was designed to be doable. In the end, you'll have developed some essential cooking skills, found some fantastic go-to recipes, and improved your health.

EASY, HEALTHY RECIPES

The recipes in the book are healthy but also easy. In fact, many of these recipes were developed while I was cooking on the fly for my family. Even as a food blogger and dietitian, I still get overwhelmed trying to get dinner on the table, so the recipes in this book use everyday, inexpensive ingredients. Many of them fit into an "easy" category, such as 5-ingredient, 30 minutes or less, one pot/pan/bowl, sheet pan, or no-cook. I also provide dietary labels, such as vegan, vegetarian, gluten-free, nut-free, and dairy-free, where applicable, so you can quickly scan the recipes if you or someone in your family has special dietary needs.

In addition to the recipes in the plan, you'll find delicious bonus recipes in chapter 8 that will help you continue your healthy lifestyle beyond the 30-day plan.

PRACTICAL TIPS AND SHORTCUTS

To make cooking easier, try a few of these shortcuts:

1. **Prep and wash everything as soon as you get home.** If anything needs to be washed and prepped for the week, do it as you are putting groceries away, so you make sure it gets done. For instance, did you buy strawberries for a snack? Great! Wash and cut them up the way you like them. Check the recipes and see what other prep work can be done right away. It makes it so much easier when it comes time to cook.

2. **Consider batch-cooking grains.** I often batch-cook grains such as quinoa and freeze half. That way the next time I need cooked quinoa, it's already done.

3. **Consider making two meals in one night.** If you have one night that is going to be super busy, cook meals for two nights the day before, so your next day's meal is ready and waiting for you. Or make a double batch and plan to eat leftovers.

Step Four: End Mindless Eating

Mindless eating is eating without paying attention to your food or how or why you are eating (actual hunger, emotions, limited time, or something else?). This is something I work on with every client I've ever had. It's easy to fall into a habit (or a trap) of eating mindlessly, and I don't want you to undermine the hard work of cooking all this healthy food by doing that.

The opposite of mindless eating is mindful eating, which just means being aware of your hunger levels and honoring them. Research shows that learning mindful eating techniques supports a healthy weight loss program. It sounds simple to eat only when you are hungry and stop when you're full, but because of cultural norms we learned as children, such as having to clean our plate, we all often overeat without even knowing it. Going on diets that restrict eating, and paying less attention to our food, just makes things worse. Here are some simple steps to becoming a more mindful eater:

1. Label your hunger on a scale of 1 to 10 before you sit down to eat. Aim to be between a 4 and a 7 level of hunger when you eat.

2. Eat until you are 80 percent full and no longer feel hungry. Do not stuff yourself.

3. Remove any distractions, such as phones, TVs, and books. And don't drive while you eat. When you eat, just eat.

Step Five: **Sleep, Relax, and Exercise**

Use a healthy lifestyle to maximize the effects of your 30-day plan. Sleep, relaxation, and exercise make all the difference when it comes to the success of your 30-day plan.

SLEEP

If I had to pick between you getting enough sleep and eating healthy, I'd pick the sleep. Why? Because you are unlikely to eat well if you aren't getting enough sleep. Sleep is rejuvenating, energizing, and all-powerful. Lack of sleep skyrockets stress hormones in the body, making you crave unhealthy junk foods, caffeine, and sugar. Not having enough sleep will always lead you to eat less healthy. So if you fix the sleep, you can fix the food.

RELAX

As I mentioned earlier, when stress hormones start to rise, so do cravings for less healthy foods. I've had clients who were so stressed out about losing weight, they were preventing their weight loss! Once they removed the stress component, they started shedding weight.

Let's face it: You can't always control what stresses you in life. However, if you take just a few minutes to read, meditate, do nothing, take a bubble bath, or whatever triggers a relaxation response, you'll also stop the stress hormone cascade. Small moments of relaxation can do wonders for the results you get and how easy you find it to stick to the challenge of this 30-day plan.

EXERCISE

Everyone has a different starting fitness level. It doesn't matter if you've been intensely exercising or if you are just getting started. Any level of exercise counts, and any level of progress counts. Since becoming a mom, my own workouts are 30 minutes or less. Regardless of where you begin, including exercise in your 30-day program is extremely important for optimal results. Read through chapter 2 for the best way to set up your week for the best outcome. Remember, getting started is the hardest part, but you'll feel great after that first workout.

Once you've completed these five steps, congrats! It's time to get started on your 30-day plan.

PART TWO

YOUR 30-DAY WEIGHT LOSS PLAN

This 30-day plan was curated with you in mind. Whether you follow it exactly or modify it to fit your life, it's meant to put you on the path to successfully achieve your health goals. Let's get started!

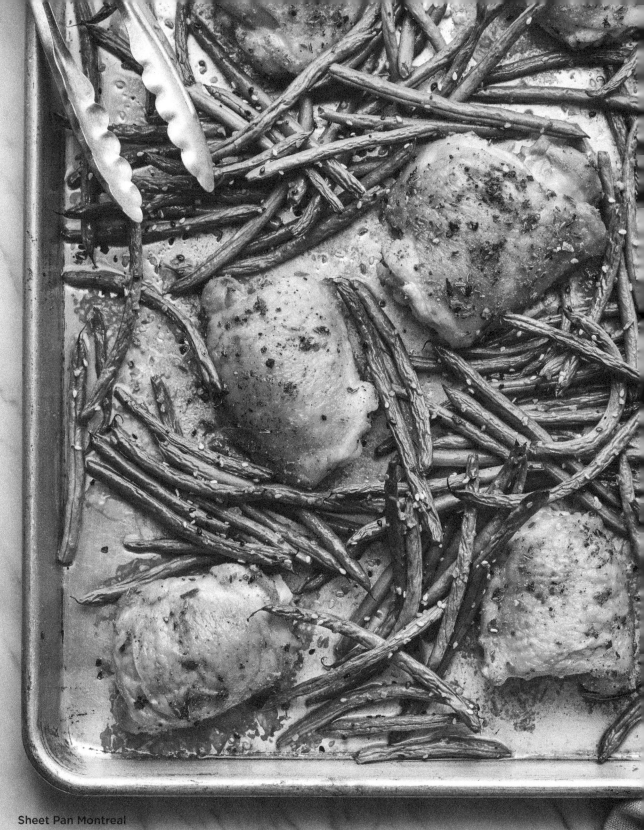

Sheet Pan Montreal
Chicken and Everything
Green Beans, page 59

CHAPTER 4

Meal Plan for Days 1 to 7

CONGRATS ON STARTING THE FIRST WEEK OF YOUR 30-DAY PLAN!
It's going to be a great week filled with flavorful food, sweaty workouts, and the beginning to a new, slimmer you. If you feel overwhelmed this week, understand that is 100 percent normal. Soon, you'll be a pro—it just takes a little practice in the kitchen and in the gym. Getting started is the hardest part, and you've already done that, so let's knock it out of the park together!

Your Workouts

Here is a blank chart to plan your workouts for the week based on what you learned in chapter 2. Start *easy* this week. If you are a regular exerciser, try for five days of workouts this week (three cardio workouts and two strength training and stretching days) and two rest days. If you are new to exercise, try to work out three days this week (two or three days of cardio and three days of strength training—and you can combine them into three workouts if you are exercising only three days a week) and see how you feel.

SUNDAY	MONDAY	TUESDAY	WEDNESDAY	THURSDAY	FRIDAY	SATURDAY

In the chart, fill in what days you rested and what days you worked out, the type of workout, and how long you exercised. Here's a sample chart. Remember, yours may or may not look like this. Make an exercise plan for where you are starting now.

SUNDAY	MONDAY	TUESDAY	WEDNESDAY	THURSDAY	FRIDAY	SATURDAY
LISS cardio: 30 minutes Stretching or foam rolling: 10 minutes	Full-body strength training: 30 minutes Stretching or foam rolling: 10 minutes	Rest/active recovery: walk, stretch, or light yoga	Full-body strength training: 30 minutes Optional stretching or foam rolling: 10 minutes	HIIT cardio: 20 minutes	Strength and cardio: 30–45 minutes Stretching or foam rolling: 10 minutes	Rest/active recovery: walk, stretch, or light yoga

Your Habit Tracker

Use this chart to help keep yourself accountable for your SMART goals by breaking your big goals into smaller ones. I've added an example on the first line.

HABIT	SUN	M	T	W	TH	F	SAT
Drink 8 glasses of water	X		X			X	X

Meal Plan

WEEK 1	SUN (Daily calories: 1,567)	M (Daily calories: 1,540)	T (Daily calories: 1,769)	W (Daily calories: 1,641)	TH (Daily calories: 1,806)	F (Daily calories: 1,644)	SAT (Daily calories: 1,496)
Breakfast	Power Chocolate Peanut Butter Protein Smoothie (2 servings) (page 70)	Cheesy Cauliflower Rice Quiche (page 53)	Blueberry Collagen Oatmeal Bake (page 58)	Cheesy Cauliflower Rice Quiche (leftovers)	Blueberry Collagen Oatmeal Bake (leftovers)	Chocolate Chip Cookie Dough Overnight Oats (page 63)	Chocolate Chip Cookie Dough Overnight Oats (leftovers)
Lunch	Bento Boxes (page 71)	Not Your Average BLT (page 54)	Not Your Average BLT (leftovers)	Blackened Cod and Parmesan Zucchini Slices (leftovers)	Sheet Pan Montreal Chicken and Everything Green Beans (leftovers)	Creamy Chickpea and Avocado Lettuce Wraps (page 64)	Creamy Chickpea and Avocado Lettuce Wraps (leftovers)
Dinner	Veggie Sourdough Pizzas (leftovers)	Blackened Cod and Parmesan Zucchini Slices (page 56)	Sheet Pan Montreal Chicken and Everything Green Beans (page 59)	Easy Beef Tostadas and Cilantro Lime Cauliflower Rice (page 60)	Easy Beef Tostadas and Cilantro Lime Cauliflower Rice (leftovers)	Tofu Peanut Ramen Stir-Fry (page 65)	Veggie Sourdough Pizzas (page 67)
Dessert	Black Bean Brownies (leftovers)	Black Bean Brownies (page 57)	Black Bean Brownies (leftovers)	Black Bean Brownies (leftovers)	Black Bean Brownies (leftovers)	Black Bean Brownies (leftovers)	Black Bean Brownies (leftovers)

Shopping List

Here is your shopping list for the week. Make sure to check out the recipes before heading to the store. If you choose to make substitutions in your recipes, you'll need to update the shopping list. Check your pantry to make sure you don't buy double of any ingredients, especially spices, that you might already have on hand.

Fresh Produce

- → Avocado (1)
- → Bananas (2)
- → Basil leaves, fresh (1 bunch)
- → Cabbage, green (1 head)
- → Carrots (2)
- → Carrots, baby, 1 (2-pound) bag
- → Celery (3 bunches)
- → Cilantro, fresh (1 bunch)
- → Garlic (2 heads)
- → Grapes (4 cups)

- → Green beans (2 pounds)
- → Lemon (1)
- → Lettuce, butter (1 head)
- → Lettuce, romaine (1 bunch)
- → Lime (1)
- → Mixed greens (4 cups)
- → Onions, white (2)
- → Parsley, fresh (1 bunch)

- → Pepper, jalapeño (1)
- → Peppers, mini (1 pound)
- → Scallions (2)
- → Spinach, baby (1 bunch)
- → Tomato, large (1)
- → Tomatoes, cherry (3 pints)
- → Tomatoes, Roma (6)
- → Zucchini (6)

Frozen

- → Blueberries, frozen, 1 (10-ounce) bag
- → Cauliflower, frozen, 1 (12-ounce) bag

- → Cauliflower rice, 1 (24-ounce bag)

- → Vegetables, frozen stir-fry mix, 1 (1-pound) bag

Pantry

- → Almond butter
- → Artichokes, packed in water, 1 (12-ounce) jar
- → Baking powder
- → Basil, dried
- → Beans, black, 1 (15-ounce) can
- → Beans, refried, 1 (15-ounce) can

- → Cajun seasoning
- → Cashew butter
- → Chia seeds
- → Chickpeas, 3 (15-ounce) cans
- → Chocolate chips, mini
- → Chocolate chips, semisweet
- → Cilantro, dried

- → Cinnamon
- → Cocoa powder, unsweetened
- → Coconut aminos or soy sauce
- → Collagen powder
- → Crackers, whole-grain, 1 (9-ounce) box

- Everything bagel seasoning
- Garlic powder
- Garlic salt
- Ginger, ground
- Maple syrup
- Mayonnaise, avocado oil
- Montreal seasoning
- Mustard, Dijon
- Mustard, yellow
- Nonstick cooking spray
- Oats, rolled
- Oil, avocado
- Oil, coconut
- Oil, extra-virgin olive
- Oil, sesame
- Olives, pitted and sliced black, 1 (4-ounce) can
- Onion flakes
- Onion powder
- Oregano, dried
- Paprika, smoked
- Peanut butter, creamy
- Pepper, black
- Protein powder, chocolate
- Protein powder, vanilla
- Ramen noodles, gluten-free brown rice, 1 (8-ounce) package
- Salt, flaky
- Salt, garlic
- Salt, sea
- Sriracha
- Stevia drops
- Sugar, coconut or brown
- Sun-dried tomatoes, 1 (8-ounce) jar
- Taco seasoning
- Tahini
- Thyme, dried
- Tomatoes, diced, 2 (15-ounce) cans
- Vanilla extract
- Vinegar, rice

Refrigerated
- Beef, 90 percent lean ground (1 pound)
- Bread, whole-grain (1 loaf)
- Bread, whole-wheat sourdough (1 loaf)
- Cheese, Cheddar, sliced (4 ounces)
- Cheese, Cheddar, shredded, 1 (8-ounce) package
- Cheese, Mexican, shredded, 1 (8-ounce) package
- Cheese, mozzarella, shredded, 1 (8-ounce) package
- Cheese, Parmesan, grated, 1 (5-ounce) container
- Chicken thighs, bone-in, (3 pounds)
- Cod fillets (4)
- Corn tortillas, 8 (6-inch)
- Eggs (11)
- Hummus (omit if you make Roasted Garlic Hummus, page 87)
- Milk, unsweetened almond or other unsweetened (1 gallon)
- Tempeh (1 pound)
- Tofu, extra-firm or high-protein (1 pound)
- Turkey deli meat, nitrate-free (8 ounces)

Cheesy Cauliflower Rice Quiche

Gluten-free, Nut-free, Vegetarian
SERVES 4 | **PREP TIME:** 10 minutes | **COOK TIME:** 30 minutes

This lightened-up, healthy cauliflower quiche is full of cheesy deliciousness without all the calories of a typical quiche. It's simple to make, and you'll love the big flavor.

- **1 tablespoon avocado oil, plus more to grease the baking dish**
- **12 ounces frozen cauliflower rice** (see Substitution Tip)
- **8 eggs**
- **¼ teaspoon sea salt**
- **¼ teaspoon black pepper**
- **¼ teaspoon garlic powder**
- **¼ teaspoon onion powder**
- **½ cup shredded sharp Cheddar cheese**

1. Preheat the oven to 375°F. Grease an 8-by-8-inch baking dish with avocado oil.

2. Put 1 tablespoon of avocado oil in a large nonstick skillet. Break up the frozen cauliflower rice as much as possible; then add it to the pan. Cook on medium-high heat for 10 minutes or until the cauliflower rice is fully defrosted and slightly softened; then remove from the heat.

3. In a large bowl, whisk the eggs, salt, pepper, garlic powder, and onion powder.

4. Spread the cauliflower rice in an even layer in the baking dish, followed by the eggs. Top with the cheese. Bake for 30 minutes, or until the eggs are fully set. Serve.

> SUBSTITUTION TIP: **Feel free to substitute 1 cup of any finely chopped vegetable, such as broccoli, bell peppers, or spinach, for the cauliflower rice, for a different spin on this delicious recipe.**

Per Serving: Calories: 238; Fat: 18g; Carbohydrates: 3g; Fiber: 1g; Protein: 17g; Sodium: 387mg

Not Your Average BLT

Dairy-free, Nut-free, Vegan
SERVES 4 | **PREP TIME:** 15 minutes | **COOK TIME:** 20 minutes

Tempeh is a cultured soy and grain product that is high in protein. And since it's fermented, it's rich in prebiotic fiber, which feeds the good bacteria in your GI tract and may aid in digestive health and decrease inflammation. Substituting tempeh for bacon in this spin on the BLT is a delicious way to include this healthy food in your diet.

½ **cup soy sauce or coconut aminos**

1 **teaspoon garlic powder**

1 **teaspoon smoked paprika**

¾ **teaspoon maple syrup**

2 **tablespoons sesame oil, divided**

1 **pound tempeh, cut into ¼-inch slices, divided** (see Substitution Tip)

2 **tablespoons avocado oil mayonnaise, divided**

8 **slices thin-sliced whole-grain bread, divided**

2 **tablespoons yellow mustard, divided**

1 **large tomato, sliced**

8 **romaine lettuce leaves**

SIDE DISH

4 **cups baby carrots**

1. In a small bowl, combine the soy sauce, garlic powder, paprika, and maple syrup to make a sauce.

2. Heat 1 tablespoon of sesame oil in a large nonstick skillet over medium-high heat. Add about half the tempeh slices and cook, flipping once, until both sides are golden brown, 3 to 5 minutes on each side.

3. When the first batch of tempeh is done, add half the sauce to the pan with the cooked tempeh and continue cooking until no liquid remains, coating the tempeh as you cook. Remove the first batch of tempeh and sauce from the pan and set aside.

4. Repeat steps 2 and 3 with the remaining tempeh and sauce.

5. Spread ½ tablespoon of mayonnaise each on four slices of bread. On the other four slices, spread ½ tablespoon mustard on each.

6. Assemble each sandwich with one-quarter of the tempeh bacon, two slices of tomato, and two lettuce leaves between one slice of bread with mayo and one slice of bread with mustard.

7. Serve with a side of 1 cup of baby carrots per person.

SUBSTITUTION TIP: **You could also use turkey bacon instead of tempeh in this recipe and skip the sauce.**

Per Serving: Calories: 594; Fat: 28g; Carbohydrates: 66g; Fiber: 11g; Protein: 30g; Sodium: 639mg

Blackened Cod and Parmesan Zucchini Slices

30 minutes or less, 5-ingredient, Gluten-free, Nut-free, Sheet pan
SERVES 4 | **PREP TIME:** 10 minutes | **COOK TIME:** 20 minutes

This easy two-sheet-pan meal introduces juicy and flaky cod blackened with a flavorful blend of Cajun seasoning and roasted to perfection. Served with a side of cheesy roasted zucchini slices, this delicious meal has the added bonus of easy cleanup. Feel free to use any summer squash in place of zucchini.

Nonstick cooking spray

4 cod fillets (2 pounds total)

2 teaspoons Cajun seasoning

4 zucchini, cut into ¼-inch rounds

¼ teaspoon garlic salt

¼ teaspoon freshly ground black pepper

¼ cup grated Parmesan cheese

1. Preheat the oven to 400°F. Line two baking sheets with aluminum foil and spray with nonstick cooking spray. Place one rack in the top of the oven and one in the bottom.

2. Dry the cod pieces with a paper towel and rub them with the Cajun seasoning. Evenly spread the seasoned cod on one baking sheet. Place the baking sheet with the fish on the bottom rack of the oven and roast for 20 minutes, or until the fish is flaky and reaches an internal temperature of 145°F.

3. While the fish is cooking, evenly spread the zucchini rounds on the other baking sheet. Spray the tops of the rounds with nonstick cooking spray and then sprinkle them with the garlic salt, pepper, and Parmesan cheese. Place that baking sheet on the top rack of the oven and bake for 15 minutes, or until the zucchini is soft and golden brown. Serve immediately.

PERFECTLY HEALTHY: **Cod is high in protein and low in fat. It has a mild taste and a hearty texture, making it as versatile as it is delicious. It's also a good source of phosphorus, niacin, and vitamin B$_{12}$.**

Per Serving: Calories: 244; Fat: 4g; Carbohydrates: 7g; Fiber: 2g; Protein: 45g; Sodium: 381mg

Black Bean Brownies

Dairy-free, Gluten-free, Vegetarian
SERVES 9 | **PREP TIME:** 10 minutes | **COOK TIME:** 30 minutes

These brownies are rich and decadent—and you'd never guess the secret ingredient if you didn't read the title of the recipe. I remember the first time I heard about making desserts out of beans, I was skeptical to say the least. But these fudgy, chocolaty brownies will convert you to a bean-based dessert fan too!

1 (15-ounce) can black beans, drained and rinsed

½ cup unsweetened cocoa powder

½ cup coconut sugar or brown sugar

¼ cup almond butter
(see Substitution Tip)

2 eggs

1 teaspoon vanilla extract

½ teaspoon baking powder

¼ teaspoon sea salt

½ cup semisweet chocolate chips

1. Preheat the oven to 350°F. Line an 8-by-8-inch baking dish with parchment paper.

2. In a food processor, blend together the black beans, cocoa powder, coconut sugar, almond butter, eggs, vanilla, baking powder, and salt. When everything is blended smoothly, fold in the chocolate chips.

3. Pour the batter into the baking dish and bake for 25 to 30 minutes, until a toothpick inserted in the center comes out clean. Let cool completely for at least 1 hour before cutting them into nine squares. These brownies can be enjoyed warm or cold.

SUBSTITUTION TIP: **You can substitute cashew butter for almond butter if you don't love almonds or just want a slightly different flavor.**

LEFTOVER TIP: **You can refrigerate leftovers for up to 1 week.**

Per Serving: Calories: 210; Fat: 9g; Carbohydrates: 30g; Fiber: 7g; Protein: 8g; Sodium: 110mg

Blueberry Collagen Oatmeal Bake

Gluten-free, One bowl, Vegetarian
SERVES 4 | **PREP TIME:** 10 minutes | **COOK TIME:** 45 minutes

I love oatmeal, but I don't love feeling hungry five seconds after I'm done eating it. A warm bowl of this cinnamon-baked oatmeal, bursting with warm berries and packed with protein, is sure to keep you full and satisfied all morning long! For even more protein, top each serving with 1 tablespoon of peanut butter or almond butter.

- 2 tablespoons coconut oil, melted, plus more to grease the baking dish
- 2 cups rolled oats
- ¾ cup collagen powder
- 2 teaspoons cinnamon
- 1 teaspoon baking powder
- ¼ teaspoon sea salt
- 1½ cups unsweetened almond milk or other unsweetened milk
- 2 tablespoons maple syrup
- 1 egg
- 1 teaspoon vanilla extract
- 1½ cups frozen blueberries

1. Preheat the oven to 375°F. Grease an 8-by-8-inch baking dish with coconut oil.

2. In a large bowl, combine the oats, collagen, cinnamon, baking powder, and salt.

3. Add the milk, melted coconut oil, maple syrup, egg, and vanilla. Mix well. Fold in the blueberries and gently mix until combined.

4. Pour the mixture into the baking dish and bake for 45 minutes, or until set. Serve.

PERFECTLY HEALTHY: Collagen is an essential component in protecting our joints and the elasticity of our skin. Collagen powder is made from animal tissue, and eating it can help replenish amino acids that are needed to repair the connective tissues in our body. You can find it online or at most major grocery stores in the protein powder section or supplement section. If you don't want to use collagen powder, egg white protein powder makes a great substitute.

Per Serving: Calories: 365; Fat: 12g; Carbohydrates: 43g; Fiber: 7g; Protein: 23g; Sodium: 387mg

Sheet Pan Montreal Chicken and Everything Green Beans

5-ingredient, Dairy-free, Gluten-free, Nut-free, Sheet pan
SERVES 4 | **PREP TIME:** 10 minutes | **COOK TIME:** 45 minutes

Montreal seasoning is a flavorful mix of garlic, coriander, dill, black pepper, red pepper flakes, salt, and pepper. Traditionally used for steak, it gives a surprising burst of flavor to crispy chicken thighs. This juicy, flavorful chicken is served with everything green beans for another easy double sheet pan meal!

Nonstick cooking spray

3 pounds bone-in, skin-on chicken thighs (see Substitution Tip)

¾ teaspoon Montreal seasoning

6 cups green beans, trimmed

½ teaspoon sea salt

1 teaspoon everything bagel seasoning (see Cooking Tip)

1. Preheat the oven to 425°F. Line two baking sheets with aluminum foil and spray with nonstick cooking spray. Place one rack in the top of the oven and one in the bottom.

2. Coat the chicken thighs with the Montreal seasoning and evenly spread them on one baking sheet. Place the pan on the bottom rack of the oven and bake for 40 to 45 minutes, or until the chicken reaches an internal temperature of 165°F.

3. Spread the green beans on the second baking sheet and spray with nonstick cooking spray; then sprinkle with the salt and everything bagel seasoning. Bake for 20 to 25 minutes, until fork-tender and slightly browned on the edges. Serve immediately.

SUBSTITUTION TIP: **You can use 2 pounds of boneless, skinless chicken thighs instead of bone-in.**

COOKING TIP: **Everything bagel seasoning is available online and at many grocery stores, but if you can't find it, you can make your own. Combine ¼ teaspoon of poppy seeds, ⅛ teaspoon of white sesame seeds, ⅛ teaspoon of black sesame seeds, ⅛ teaspoon of minced dried garlic, ⅛ teaspoon of minced dried onion, and ⅛ teaspoon of flaky sea salt.**

Per Serving: Calories: 441; Fat: 14g; Carbohydrates: 10g; Fiber: 4g; Protein: 70g; Sodium: 691mg

Easy Beef Tostadas and Cilantro Lime Cauliflower Rice

Gluten-free, Nut-free

SERVES 4 | **PREP TIME:** 5 minutes | **COOK TIME:** 40 minutes

In this recipe, everybody gets to assemble their own tostadas, which is always fun. Served with fresh cilantro lime cauliflower rice, this meal makes for a real fiesta.

FOR THE TOSTADAS

Nonstick cooking spray

½ tablespoon
avocado oil

½ white onion, chopped

2 garlic cloves, minced

1 pound 90 percent
lean ground beef
(see Substitution Tip)

¼ cup taco seasoning

8 (6-inch) corn tortillas

1 (15-ounce) can diced
tomatoes, drained

1 (15-ounce) can
refried beans

1 cup shredded
Mexican cheese

2 cups shredded
cabbage

Chopped scallions, for
garnish (optional)

Fresh Homemade Salsa,
for garnish (optional;
page 62)

FOR THE CILANTRO LIME
CAULIFLOWER RICE

1 tablespoon avocado oil

12 ounces frozen or
fresh cauliflower rice

1 teaspoon dried
cilantro or
1 tablespoon chopped
fresh cilantro

1 teaspoon taco
seasoning

Juice of ½ lime
(2 tablespoons)

Sea salt

Freshly ground
black pepper

TO MAKE THE TOSTADAS

1. Preheat the oven to 400°F. Line a baking sheet with aluminum foil and spray with nonstick cooking spray.

2. Heat the avocado oil in a large nonstick skillet over medium-high heat. Add the onion and garlic and cook for 1 to 2 minutes, until the onion is translucent and tender. Add the ground beef to the skillet, mix in the taco seasoning, and cook until browned, about 10 minutes.

3. While the meat is cooking, spread the tortillas on the baking sheet and spray the tops with cooking oil. Bake for 5 minutes; then flip and bake for another 5 minutes. Flip one more time and bake for another 3 to 5 minutes, or until they are as crisp as you like.

4. When the beef is browned, add the diced tomatoes. Cook until the liquid evaporates, about 5 minutes.

5. To assemble the tostadas, spread each baked tortilla with ¼ cup of refried beans, about 2 tablespoons of the meat mixture, 2 tablespoons of cheese, and ¼ cup of cabbage. Garnish with scallions and serve with salsa, if desired.

TO MAKE THE CILANTRO LIME CAULIFLOWER RICE

6. In a large nonstick skillet over medium-high heat, combine the oil and cauliflower rice. Toss to break up and separate the rice.

7. Add the cilantro, taco seasoning, and lime juice and stir to combine. Leave the cauliflower rice to cook without stirring for 5 to 8 minutes to create a crunchy layer underneath. Season with salt and pepper. Serve about ½ cup of cauliflower rice with two tostadas per serving.

SUBSTITUTION TIP: **Feel free to substitute ground turkey or chicken for beef in this recipe.**

LEFTOVER TIP: **Store the beef mixture separately from the tostadas so the tostadas stay crispy. After they've cooled completely, store the baked tostadas in the pantry for up to a week. Store the ground beef and cauliflower rice separately for up to 5 days in the refrigerator.**

Per Serving (without the Fresh Homemade Salsa)**:** Calories: 790; Fat: 43g; Carbohydrates: 53g; Fiber: 7g; Protein: 47g; Sodium: 856mg

Fresh Homemade Salsa

30 minutes or less, Dairy-free, Gluten-free, No-cook, Nut-free, Vegan
MAKES: about 4 cups | **PREP TIME:** 15 minutes

Homemade salsa is so fresh and flavorful, juicy, and delicious that you'll wonder why you ever bought salsa in a jar. You can use this fresh salsa with any Southwestern-style dish, or grab some chips or cut veggies and dig in.

6 **Roma tomatoes,** quartered

½ **white onion,** roughly chopped

1 **scallion**

1 **jalapeño pepper,** seeded and deveined

¼ **cup chopped fresh** cilantro leaves

2 **tablespoons freshly** squeezed lime juice

½ **teaspoon sea salt**

1. Place the tomatoes, onion, scallion, jalapeño, cilantro, lime juice, and salt in a food processor.

2. Pulse until combined but still a little chunky, 10 to 15 times.

LEFTOVER TIP: **Store the salsa in an airtight container in the refrigerator for up to 5 days.**

Per Serving: Calories: 31; Fat: 0g; Carbohydrates: 6g; Fiber: 1g; Protein: 1g; Sodium: 152mg

Chocolate Chip Cookie Dough Overnight Oats

Gluten-free, No-cook, Vegetarian
SERVES 4 | **PREP TIME:** 5 minutes | **CHILL TIME:** 4 hours

Ever wished you could eat cookies for breakfast? These cookie dough overnight oats—with chocolate chips in every bite—are the answer to your cravings! When I made this for my hubby, he said it was the best overnight oats he'd ever had in his life. Everyone enjoys chocolate chips at breakfast!

3 cups unsweetened almond milk or other unsweetened milk, divided

2 cups rolled oats, divided

1 cup vanilla protein powder, divided (see Perfectly Healthy note)

4 tablespoons cashew butter, divided

2 tablespoons mini chocolate chips, divided

2 tablespoons maple syrup, divided

4 teaspoons chia seeds, divided

2 teaspoons vanilla extract, divided

1. In each of four mason jars (or resealable containers), combine ¾ cup of milk, ½ cup of oats, ¼ cup of vanilla protein powder, 1 tablespoon of cashew butter, 1½ teaspoons of mini chocolate chips, ½ tablespoon of maple syrup, 1 teaspoon of chia seeds, and ½ teaspoon of vanilla. Mix the ingredients in each mason jar well.

2. Place the jars in the refrigerator for at least 4 hours and up to 5 days. Enjoy cold.

Cooking Tip: Not in love with the idea of cold oats? After they've "cooked" in the refrigerator, heat them up in the microwave—but be sure to save the chocolate chips and add them *after* you heat the oats.

PERFECTLY HEALTHY: You can find protein powder near the protein bars in the grocery store. I recommend whey protein for dairy lovers and pea protein for my dairy-free friends. Look for something with only ingredients you can pronounce and less than 10 grams of carbohydrates per serving.

Per Serving: Calories: 318; Fat 8g; Carbohydrates: 37g; Fiber: 6g; Protein: 25g; Sodium: 100mg

Creamy Chickpea and Avocado Lettuce Wraps

30 minutes or less, Dairy-free, No-cook, Nut-free, Vegetarian
SERVES 4 | **PREP TIME:** 15 minutes

I'm always looking for new ways to sneak beans into my diet because on their own they aren't my favorite food. This recipe replaces canned tuna or chicken with canned chickpeas mixed with creamy avocado, fresh seasonings, and crunchy veggies inside a cool, crisp lettuce wrap. While I would typically put this mixture on a sandwich, my mother-in-law suggested eating it in lettuce wraps, and I was blown away by how delicious it is.

1 (15-ounce) can chickpeas, drained and rinsed

1 avocado

1 teaspoon lemon juice

⅓ cup chopped fresh parsley

1 teaspoon garlic powder

1 teaspoon sea salt

½ teaspoon freshly ground black pepper

¼ cup chopped white onion

4 celery stalks, chopped

2 large carrots, chopped

8 butter lettuce leaves

SIDE DISHES

4 cups mini sweet peppers

4 cups grapes

1. In a large bowl, use a fork or a potato masher to mash together the chickpeas and avocado. Mix in the lemon juice, parsley, garlic powder, salt, and pepper. Then stir in the onion, celery, and carrots.

2. Divide the bean mixture onto the lettuce leaves and gently wrap each portion.

3. Serve two filled lettuce leaves with a side of 1 cup of mini sweet peppers and 1 cup of grapes per person.

LEFTOVER TIP: Store the remaining chickpea and avocado mixture separately from the lettuce leaves and assemble when you're ready to eat.

SUBSTITUTION TIP: As I mentioned, you could also eat this in a sandwich on thin-sliced bread. This would add about 140 calories, though, so make sure to account for that (and add bread to your grocery list).

Per Serving: Calories: 316; Fat: 10g; Carbohydrates: 52g; Fiber: 13g; Protein: 10g; Sodium: 656mg

Tofu Peanut Ramen Stir-Fry

30 minutes or less, 5-ingredient, Dairy-free, Gluten-free, Vegan
SERVES 4 | **PREP TIME:** 5 minutes | **COOK TIME:** 20 minutes

One of my go-to meals is this easy stir-fry with a homemade peanut sauce. This flavorful meal comes together in less than 30 minutes and will be a crowd-pleaser. Brown rice ramen is turning up in more and more grocery stores, but if you can't find it, just use brown rice.

2 tablespoons sesame oil, divided

1 pound extra-firm high-protein tofu, cubed (see Substitution and Cooking Tips)

4 cups frozen stir-fry vegetables

2 cups gluten-free brown rice ramen noodles (see Substitution Tip)

¾ cup Easy Peanut Sauce (page 66)

1. In a large nonstick skillet, heat 1 tablespoon of sesame oil and pan-fry the tofu until golden brown and crispy all over. Remove from the pan and set aside.

2. In the same skillet, heat the remaining 1 tablespoon of oil and the vegetables. Cover and cook for 10 to 12 minutes, stirring occasionally, until the vegetables are soft.

3. Meanwhile, in a medium pot, cook the noodles according to the package directions.

4. When the veggies are ready, add the tofu, noodles, and peanut sauce to the skillet. Mix well and serve.

SUBSTITUTION TIP: **This recipe is very customizable. You can substitute any type of protein for the tofu. Consider 1 pound of shrimp, chicken cut into strips, or flank steak strips. Also, you can substitute brown rice or quinoa for the ramen noodles.**

COOKING TIP: **High-protein tofu is already pressed and ready to go. It's available at Trader Joe's along with some other health and natural food stores. If you can't find it, you can make your own. Get 30 ounces of extra-firm tofu and press it to get 16 ounces of high-protein tofu. To press your tofu, place a dish towel on a flat plate, and put the block of tofu on it, followed by another dish towel and some heavy pots and pans. Let it press and drain for 30 minutes.**

Per Serving (with Easy Peanut Sauce): Calories: 518; Fat: 25g; Carbohydrates: 48g; Fiber: 5g; Protein: 26g; Sodium: 423mg

Easy Peanut Sauce

30 minutes or less, Dairy-free, Gluten-free, No-cook, One bowl, Vegan
MAKES: about ¾ cup | **PREP TIME:** 5 minutes

If you thought that peanut sauce was something you can get only at a restaurant, think again. It's so easy to make, it can be a staple in your home. This rich, creamy peanut sauce is versatile as a dipping sauce, a go-to stir-fry sauce, or even a salad dressing when thinned with water.

¼ **cup creamy peanut butter** (see Substitution Tip)

¼ **cup soy sauce or coconut aminos**

¼ **cup rice vinegar**

1 **tablespoon coconut sugar or brown sugar**

2 **teaspoons garlic powder**

1 **teaspoon ground ginger**

1 **tablespoon sriracha** (optional)

Combine the peanut butter, soy sauce, vinegar, sugar, garlic powder, ginger, and sriracha in a medium bowl. Mix well.

LEFTOVER TIP: **This peanut sauce stays fresh for 3 to 5 days in the refrigerator.**

SUBSTITUTION TIP: **You can substitute cashew butter or almond butter for the peanut butter if you don't tolerate peanuts or just want a slightly different flavor.**

Per Serving: Calories: 130; Fat: 8g; Carbohydrates: 11g; Fiber: 1g; Protein: 4g; Sodium: 377mg

Veggie Sourdough Pizzas

30 minutes or less, Nut-free, Sheet pan, Vegetarian
SERVES 4 | **PREP TIME:** 10 minutes | **COOK TIME:** 15 minutes

Wait, can you eat pizza on a weight loss plan? Heck yes! These sourdough pizzas amp up the flavor with homemade sauce, flavorful whole-grain sourdough bread, and veggie toppings for a pizza night that's as good for you as it tastes.

Nonstick cooking spray

8 thick slices whole-wheat sourdough bread (see Substitution Tip)

1 cup Easy Blender Pizza Sauce (page 68), divided

1 cup baby spinach, shredded, divided

1½ cups shredded mozzarella cheese, divided

⅓ cup fresh basil, shredded, divided

½ cup pitted and sliced black olives, divided

½ cup artichoke canned in water, drained and chopped, divided

½ cup chopped sun-dried tomatoes, divided

SIDE DISH

1¼ cups Simple Side Salad with 2 tablespoons simple dressing (page 69) per person

1. Preheat the oven to 375°F. Spray a pizza pan or baking sheet with nonstick cooking spray.

2. Lay out the bread slices on the baking sheet. Top each piece of bread with 2 tablespoons of sauce, 2 tablespoons of spinach, 3 tablespoons of mozzarella, a scant tablespoon of basil, 1 tablespoon of olives, 1 tablespoon of chopped artichokes, and 1 tablespoon of sun-dried tomatoes.

3. Bake the pizzas for 12 to 15 minutes, until the cheese is melted and bubbly. If you'd like, broil for another 1 to 2 minutes to brown the top—as if it came out of a pizza oven. Serve immediately.

SUBSTITUTION TIP: **No sourdough? Use any large slice of whole-wheat bread or a whole-wheat pita. A heartier bread will hold up better to all the toppings.**

Per Serving (with Easy Blender Pizza Sauce): Calories: 289; Fat: 8g; Carbohydrates: 34g; Fiber: 3g; Protein: 19g; Sodium: 816mg

Easy Blender Pizza Sauce

30 minutes or less, Dairy-free, Gluten-free, No-cook, Nut-free
MAKES: about 2 cups | **PREP TIME:** 5 minutes

This no-cook, no-fail pizza sauce is made from just a few pantry staples and can be ready in less than 5 minutes, so your pizza night won't run late.

1 (15-ounce) can diced tomatoes

2 tablespoons dried oregano

1 tablespoon dried basil

½ tablespoon dried onion flakes

½ tablespoon garlic powder

½ tablespoon dried thyme

½ tablespoon smoked paprika

½ teaspoon sea salt

½ tablespoon freshly ground black pepper

Put the tomatoes, oregano, basil, onion flakes, garlic powder, thyme, paprika, salt, and pepper in a blender and blend until smooth.

LEFTOVER TIP: Keep the leftovers in the refrigerator for up to 2 days and in the freezer for up to 3 months.

Per Serving: Calories: 23; Fat: 0g; Carbohydrates: 5g; Fiber: 1g; Protein: 1g; Sodium: 275mg

Simple Side Salad

30 minutes or less, Gluten-free, No-cook, Nut-free, Vegan
SERVES 4 | **PREP TIME:** 10 minutes

Salad dressings can be expensive and full of added preservatives and ingredients you don't need in your diet. This simple salad dressing uses ingredients you already have in your cabinet to bring your meal to life.

FOR THE SIMPLE DRESSING
⅓ cup extra-virgin olive oil

⅓ cup water

2 tablespoons vinegar (of your choice)

1 tablespoon Dijon mustard

1 tablespoon maple syrup

1 medium garlic clove, minced

Sea salt

Black pepper

FOR THE SALAD
4 cups mixed greens

1 cup cherry tomatoes

TO MAKE THE DRESSING
1. Combine the oil, water, vinegar, mustard, maple syrup, and garlic in a jar with a tight-fitting lid. Season with salt and pepper. Cover and shake vigorously to mix. This makes about 1 cup of dressing. A single serving is 2 tablespoons.

TO MAKE THE SALAD
2. In a large bowl, toss the mixed greens and tomatoes together with ½ cup of dressing.

> LEFTOVER TIP: **The dressing keeps in the refrigerator for about 3 to 5 days. The oil might separate; if it does, let it warm to room temperature and shake again to combine.**

Per Serving: Calories: 113; Fat: 10g; Carbohydrates: 4g; Fiber: 1g; Protein: 1g; Sodium: 41mg

Power Chocolate Peanut Butter Protein Smoothie

30 minutes or less, Gluten-free, No-cook, Vegetarian
SERVES 2 | **PREP TIME:** 10 minutes

This creamy, delicious protein shake packs a secret veggie punch that will keep you fuller for longer.

2 cups frozen cauliflower

2 zucchini, cut into chunks

2 scoops chocolate protein powder

2 frozen ripe bananas, cut into chunks

2 tablespoons creamy peanut butter (see Perfectly Healthy note)

2 cups unsweetened almond milk or other unsweetened milk

2 to 4 drops liquid stevia (optional)

Put the cauliflower, zucchini, protein powder, bananas, peanut butter, milk, and stevia (if using) in a blender and blend until creamy. Serve immediately.

PERFECTLY HEALTHY: **Peanut butter is a healthy, nutrient-dense food, but make sure to measure your portion carefully because it's also calorie-dense!**

Per Serving: Calories: 382; Fat: 13g; Carbohydrates: 46g; Fiber: 12g; Protein: 30g; Sodium: 251mg

Bento Boxes

30 minutes or less, No-cook, Nut-free
SERVES 4 | **PREP TIME:** 10 minutes

Bento boxes—the adult finger food—make the perfect fun and filling lunch when you are short on prep time but still want to eat healthy! When I first started my career as a dietitian, I was working long hours in a commission-based environment where I barely had three seconds to eat my lunch, much less eat healthy foods. This became my go-to midday meal. And since you can vary the basic recipe so many ways, you won't get bored with it.

4 slices uncured nitrate-free deli turkey meat (see Substitution Tip)

4 slices Cheddar cheese slices (see Substitution Tip)

4 cups cherry tomatoes

4 cups chopped celery

4 ounces whole-grain crackers

1 cup Roasted Garlic Hummus (page 87) **or store-bought hummus**

1. Create turkey roll-ups by wrapping each piece of turkey around a Cheddar cheese slice.

2. Place 1 cup of cherry tomatoes, 1 cup of celery, 1 ounce of crackers, and ¼ cup of hummus in each bento box or on each plate. Serve immediately.

SUBSTITUTION TIP: **You can use any chicken or ham for the deli meat and other types of cheeses for the Cheddar. Additional delicious combos are ham and Swiss, chicken and pepper Jack, or pastrami and Gouda.**

Per Serving: Calories: 485; Fat: 28g; Carbohydrates: 38g; Fiber: 7g; Protein: 25g; Sodium: 1,322mg

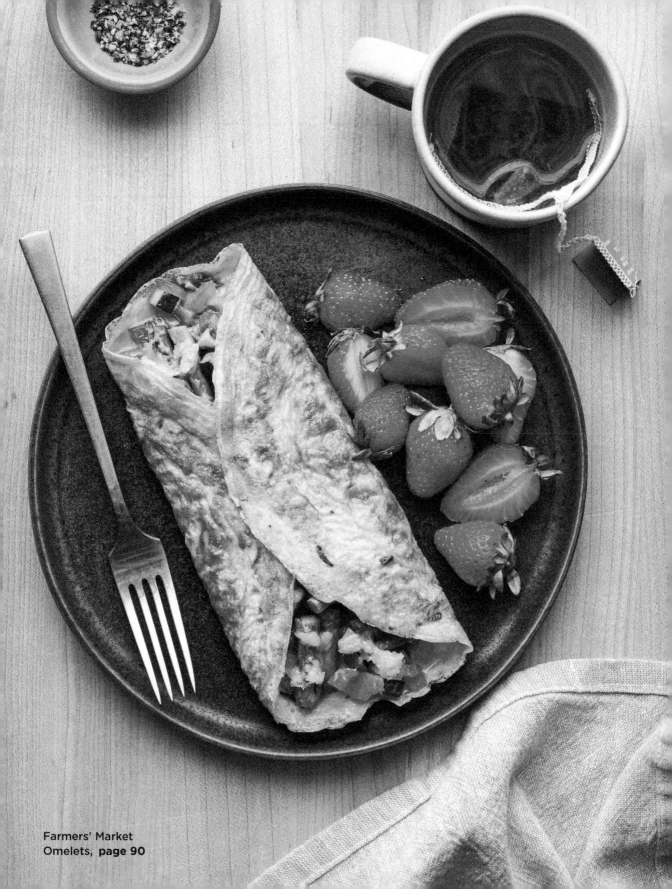

Farmers' Market
Omelets, page 90

CHAPTER 5

Meal Plan for Days 8 to 14

WELCOME TO WEEK 2 OF YOUR 30-DAY WEIGHT-LOSS PLAN. By now you should be seeing some of the success of your efforts; that will motivate you to move forward. If you don't see success right away, though, keep at it! I often have clients lose inches before they lose pounds, which isn't a bad thing. Muscle weighs more than fat, so if you are building muscle and losing fat, you are on the right track.

Your Workouts

Here is a blank chart to plan your workouts for the week based on what you learned in chapter 2.

SUNDAY	MONDAY	TUESDAY	WEDNESDAY	THURSDAY	FRIDAY	SATURDAY

Now that you've got one week down, it's time to build on your momentum just a little bit. Can you add an extra day or go for an extra walk to increase your physical activity? Plan it out in the preceding chart. Here's a sample chart.

SUNDAY	MONDAY	TUESDAY	WEDNESDAY	THURSDAY	FRIDAY	SATURDAY
LISS cardio: 30 minutes Stretching or foam rolling: 10 minutes	Full-body strength training: 30 minutes Stretching or foam rolling: 10 minutes	Rest/active recovery: walk, stretch, or light yoga	Full-body strength training: 30 minutes Optional stretching or foam rolling: 10 minutes	HIIT cardio: 20 minutes	Strength and cardio: 30–45 minutes Stretching or foam rolling: 10 minutes	Rest/active recovery: walk, stretch, or light yoga

Your Habit Tracker

Use this chart to help keep yourself accountable for your SMART goals by breaking your big goals into smaller ones.

HABIT	SUN	M	T	W	TH	F	SAT

Meal Plan

WEEK 2	SUN (Daily Calories: 1,586)	M (Daily Calories: 1,626)	T (Daily Calories: 1,630)	W (Daily Calories: 1,435)	TH (Daily Calories: 1,602)	F (Daily Calories: 1,652)	SAT (Daily Calories: 1,679)
Breakfast	Vanilla Latte Overnight Oats (2 servings) (page 92)	Blender Blueberry Greek Yogurt Pancakes (page 79)	Sweet Potato and Apple Breakfast Hash (page 83)	Blender Blueberry Greek Yogurt Pancakes (leftovers)	Sweet Potato and Apple Breakfast Hash (leftovers)	Farmers' Market Omelets (page 90)	Farmers' Market Omelets (leftovers)
Lunch	Sweet and Spicy Shrimp, Quinoa, and Asparagus (page 93)	Tofu Peanut Ramen Stir-Fry (leftovers from week 1)	Bento Boxes (leftovers from week 1)	Salmon Hummus Wraps (page 86)	Salmon Hummus Wraps (leftovers)	Roasted Veggie Buddha Bowls with Turmeric Garlic Sauce (leftovers)	Shepherd's Pie Skillet (leftovers)
Dinner	Enchilada-Stuffed Zucchini Boats (page 95)	Cheesy Tuna Quinoa Cakes (page 81)	Roasted Veggie Buddha Bowls with Turmeric Garlic Sauce (page 84)	Cheesy Tuna Quinoa Cakes (leftovers)	Shepherd's Pie Skillet (page 88)	Fried Cauliflower Rice (page 91)	Fried Cauliflower Rice (leftovers)
Dessert	Honey-Baked Pears (leftovers)	Honey-Baked Pears (page 82)	Honey-Baked Pears (leftovers)	Honey-Baked Pears (leftovers)	Honey-Baked Pears (leftovers)	Honey-Baked Pears (leftovers)	Honey-Baked Pears (leftovers)

Shopping List

Here is your shopping list for the week. Make sure to check out the recipes before heading to the store. If you choose to make substitutions in your recipes, you'll need to update the shopping list. Check your pantry to make sure you don't buy double of any ingredients, especially spices, that you might already have on hand.

Fresh Produce

→ Apples (2)
→ Asparagus (2½ pounds)
→ Broccoli (1 large head)
→ Carrots (1 pound)
→ Cauliflower (2 heads)
→ Celery (1 bunch)
→ Cilantro, fresh (1 bunch), if making Fresh Homemade Salsa (page 62)
→ Garlic (3 heads)
→ Lemons (2)
→ Lettuce, romaine (1 head)
→ Lime (1), if making Fresh Homemade Salsa (page 62)
→ Onion, red (1)
→ Onions, white (2)
→ Onions, yellow (2)
→ Pears (4)
→ Peppers, bell, any color (4), red (1)
→ Pepper, jalapeño (1), if making Fresh Homemade Salsa (page 62)
→ Potatoes, russet (2)
→ Scallions (1 bunch)
→ Spinach, baby (4 cups)
→ Strawberries (2 pints)
→ Sweet potatoes (6)
→ Tomatoes, Roma (6), if making Fresh Homemade Salsa (page 62)
→ Zucchini (5)

Frozen

→ Blueberries, frozen, 1 (10-ounce) bag
→ Cauliflower rice, frozen, 1 (24-ounce) bag
→ Edamame, shelled, frozen, 1 (14-ounce) bag

Pantry

→ All-purpose flour or cornstarch
→ Almond butter, creamy unsalted
→ Baking powder
→ Basil, dried
→ Beef broth, 1 (16-ounce) carton
→ Chia seeds
→ Chickpeas, 2 (15-ounce) cans
→ Coconut aminos or soy sauce
→ Enchilada sauce, red, 1 (16-ounce) jar
→ Garlic powder
→ Honey
→ Maple syrup
→ Nonstick cooking spray
→ Oil, avocado
→ Oil, coconut
→ Oil, extra-virgin olive
→ Oil, sesame
→ Oregano, dried

- → Oyster or fish sauce
- → Paprika, smoked
- → Pepper, black
- → Pepper, cayenne
- → Protein powder, vanilla
- → Quinoa, uncooked (1 cup)

- → Oats, rolled
- → Salmon, wild, 2 (5-ounce) cans
- → Salt, sea
- → Stevia drops
- → Taco seasoning
- → Tahini
- → Tomatoes, whole, 1 (15-ounce) can

- → Tortillas, whole-wheat, 4 (10-inch)
- → Tuna, skipjack, packed in water, 1 (7-ounce) can
- → Turmeric, ground
- → Vanilla extract
- → Vinegar, white

Refrigerated
- → Butter, salted (1 stick)
- → Cheese, Cheddar, shredded, 1 (8-ounce) bag
- → Cheese, Gruyère (2 ounces)
- → Coffee, cold brew, 1 (8-ounce) can
- → Egg whites, liquid, 1 (16-ounce) carton
- → Eggs (26)

- → Flank steak (1 pound)
- → Milk, unsweetened almond or unsweetened milk of your choice (½ pint)
- → Milk, whole (½ pint)
- → Shrimp, medium (21 to 30), peeled

and deveined (1 pound)
- → Sour cream, 1 (8-ounce) tub
- → Tofu, high-protein or extra-firm (1 pound)
- → Turkey, 93 percent lean ground (1 pound)
- → Yogurt, plain Greek

Blender Blueberry Greek Yogurt Pancakes

30 minutes or less, Gluten-free, Vegetarian
SERVES 8 | **PREP TIME:** 10 minutes | **COOK TIME:** 20 minutes

If you love buttermilk pancakes, you'll love the flavor Greek yogurt adds to your pancakes. These tender, fluffy pancakes burst with warm blueberries, and the yogurt adds a dose of protein to power your morning. Feel free to substitute another berry of your choice or add the same amount of chocolate chips.

1 cup rolled oats

1 cup plain Greek yogurt

2 eggs

¼ cup milk of your choice

¼ cup Almond Butter Syrup (optional; page 80)

1½ teaspoons baking powder

1 teaspoon vanilla extract

4 to 6 drops liquid stevia (optional)

1 teaspoon avocado oil

½ cup frozen blueberries

1. In a high-powered blender, blend the oats, yogurt, eggs, milk, almond butter syrup (if using), baking powder, vanilla, and stevia. Wait 5 minutes for the mixture to thicken.

2. Heat the avocado oil in a large nonstick skillet over medium heat. Working in batches, add ¼ cup of batter to the skillet for each pancake; then sprinkle 4 or 5 blueberries on each pancake. Flip the pancakes when they start to bubble, after 2 to 3 minutes; then cook until just set on the other side, 1 to 2 minutes. Repeat with the remaining batter. Serve.

LEFTOVER TIP: These pancakes are super freezer-friendly; they'll stay fresh for up to 3 months. Just pop them right from the freezer into the toaster. Alternatively, keep them in the refrigerator for 3 to 5 days.

Per Serving (without optional Almond Butter Syrup)**:** Calories: 175; Fat: 5g; Carbohydrates: 21g; Fiber: 3g; Protein: 11g; Sodium: 631mg

Almond Butter Syrup

30 minutes or less, 5-ingredient, Gluten-free, No-cook, One-bowl, Vegetarian
MAKES: about ¼ cup | **PREP TIME:** 10 minutes

Although I love sweet foods (I'm a "I don't think frosting is sweet enough" type person), I don't love maple syrup. I much prefer a buttery, creamy, slightly sweet topping for my pancakes. This sweet, creamy almond butter syrup is perfect for pancakes, waffles, French toast, and just plain toast. Or drizzle it over fruit. For a vegan version, use vegan butter. You can also use any other nut or seed butter, including peanut butter, cashew butter, or sunflower seed butter, for a different flavor.

2 tablespoons melted unsalted creamy almond butter

2 tablespoons melted salted butter

1 tablespoon maple syrup

In a small bowl, combine the almond butter, salted butter, and maple syrup and mix well.

LEFTOVER TIP: Store leftovers in an airtight container, such as a glass mason jar, in the refrigerator. The syrup will harden a bit, so gently heat it to thin it out before serving.

Per Serving: Calories: 113; Fat: 10g; Carbohydrates: 5g; Fiber: 1g; Protein: 2g; Sodium: 2mg

Cheesy Tuna Quinoa Cakes

5-ingredient, Gluten-free, Nut-free

SERVES 4 | **PREP TIME:** 10 minutes | **COOK TIME:** 30 minutes

These tuna cakes are baked instead of fried to save time and calories; plus, they have a cheesy fiesta flair in every bite. They are also freezer-friendly, and I can't tell you how many times I've been grateful to be able to pull a few of these from the freezer for a quick, healthy lunch. So if you love them, next time make a double batch and freeze half for an emergency healthy lunch or dinner.

Nonstick cooking spray

2 cups cooked quinoa

1 (7-ounce) can skipjack tuna packed in water, drained

2 eggs

1 cup shredded Cheddar cheese

1 tablespoon taco seasoning

Fresh Homemade Salsa (optional; page 62)

SIDE DISH

4 bell peppers (any color), cut into strips

1. Preheat the oven to 350°F. Spray a 12-cup muffin tin with nonstick cooking spray.

2. In a large bowl, mix the quinoa, tuna, eggs, Cheddar cheese, and taco seasoning until well blended. Fill each muffin cup ½ to ¾ of the way with the mixture.

3. Bake for 30 minutes or until the cakes are set and golden brown on top. Let cool completely in the tin; then run a butter knife around the edges to pop them out.

4. Serve 3 cakes per person with salsa on the side (if using), along with 1 bell pepper cut into strips, for a healthy, well-balanced meal.

COOKING TIP: **For easier cleanup, I recommend using silicone muffin liners. They are reusable and make popping these cakes right out of the muffin tin a snap.**

Per Serving (without optional Fresh Homemade Salsa)**:** Calories: 277; Fat: 13g; Carbohydrates: 19g; Fiber: 3g; Protein: 22g; Sodium: 469mg

Honey-Baked Pears

5-ingredient, Dairy-free, Gluten-free, Vegetarian
SERVES 8 | **PREP TIME:** 10 minutes | **COOK TIME:** 20 minutes

These pears are roasted with honey to tender perfection with an almond butter oat streusel topping. You can bake a batch of these pears on the weekend and eat them all week for a healthy dessert. Choose pears that are firm but not under-ripe.

4 pears

Nonstick cooking spray or avocado oil

⅓ cup almond butter

¼ cup honey

10 tablespoons rolled oats

1. Preheat the oven to 350°F. Line a baking sheet with parchment paper.

2. Halve the pears vertically and scoop out the cores. Place cut-side up on the baking sheet and spray with nonstick cooking spray.

3. In a small bowl, mix the almond butter, honey, and oats. Add a spoonful of the mixture to the hollow in each pear half.

4. Bake for 20 minutes, until the pears are tender but still slightly firm.

COOKING TIP: **A spoonful of whipped cream or light ice cream tastes delicious with these pear halves.**

Per Serving: Calories: 337; Fat: 13g; Carbohydrates: 57g; Fiber: 9g; Protein: 7g; Sodium: 4mg

Sweet Potato and Apple Breakfast Hash

Dairy-free, Gluten-free, Nut-free, Vegetarian
SERVES 4 | **PREP TIME:** 10 minutes | **COOK TIME:** 30 minutes

This savory breakfast option is delectable, with its hint of sweet apples and notes of coconut oil. I love to make this recipe as a break from the normal routine. It feels so fancy when you're digging in, but it's really easy to make.

3 tablespoons coconut oil, divided

½ red onion, finely diced

2 large sweet potatoes, cut into 1-inch cubes or small wedges

¼ cup water (optional)

2 apples, cut into 1-inch cubes or small wedges

4 cups baby spinach

Sea salt

8 eggs

1. Heat 2 tablespoons of coconut oil in a large nonstick skillet over medium heat. Add the onion and sweet potato, cover, and sauté until the sweet potato is soft, about 15 minutes. If the sweet potato starts to burn, add ¼ cup of water to the skillet.

2. Add the apples and cook for 3 to 5 minutes more, until the apple chunks begin to soften. Add the spinach and sauté until just wilted, 1 to 2 minutes. Season with salt.

3. In another large nonstick skillet, add the remaining 1 tablespoon of oil and fry the eggs the way you like them. You may have to cook them in two batches.

4. Divide the hash mixture into four servings and add 2 fried eggs on top of each. Serve immediately.

> LEFTOVER TIP: **If you know you will be eating the leftovers another day, cook only the number of eggs you need for what you're eating right then. When you are ready to eat the leftover hash, fry the remaining eggs to go with it. You can also use hard-boiled eggs.**

Per Serving: Calories: 352; Fat: 20g; Carbohydrates: 29g; Fiber: 5g; Protein: 15g; Sodium: 498mg

Roasted Veggie Buddha Bowls with Turmeric Garlic Sauce

30 minutes or less, 5-ingredient, Dairy-free, Gluten-free, Nut-free, One pot, Vegan

SERVES 4 | **PREP TIME:** 10 minutes | **COOK TIME:** 20 minutes

Buddha bowls are gorgeous veggie-packed bowls full of flavor that are said to make you so full that you have a belly like a Buddha when you finish. Don't worry, you won't really get a Buddha belly. This recipe is more likely to make your belly disappear.

Nonstick cooking spray

1 pound high-protein or extra-firm tofu, cut into ½-inch pieces (see Substitution Tip)

4 cups chopped sweet potatoes

3 cups broccoli florets

3 cups cauliflower florets

½ teaspoon sea salt

½ cup Turmeric Garlic Sauce (page 85)

1. Preheat the oven to 400°F. Line two baking sheets with aluminum foil and spray with nonstick cooking spray.

2. Evenly spread the tofu, sweet potatoes, broccoli, and cauliflower on the baking sheets. Spray with nonstick cooking spray and sprinkle with the salt. Roast for 10 minutes, turn the tofu, and roast for 10 minutes more. The tofu is done when it is golden brown and crispy, and the veggies are done when they are fork-tender.

3. Divide the tofu and vegetables among four bowls and drizzle each with 1 to 2 tablespoons of Turmeric Garlic Sauce. Serve immediately.

SUBSTITUTION TIP: **The sauce for these bowls goes nicely with any type of protein. Feel free to swap the tofu for lentils, edamame, chicken, shrimp, or whatever you have on hand.**

Per Serving (with Turmeric Garlic Sauce): Calories: 456; Fat: 23g; Carbohydrates: 42g; Fiber: 9g; Protein: 24g; Sodium: 453mg

Turmeric Garlic Sauce

30 minutes or less, Gluten-free, No-cook, Vegan
MAKES: about ¾ cup | **PREP TIME:** 10 minutes

I really think what makes Buddha bowls so delicious is the sauce. No matter what veggies and protein you use, the sauce brings the bowls to life. This is one of those sauces. Turmeric is a bright yellow spice found most often in Indian cuisine. It's known for its anti-inflammatory properties and antioxidant activity in the body. It makes this delicious garlic sauce pop with color and flavor in every bite.

½ cup extra-virgin olive oil

¼ cup water

2 tablespoons white vinegar

½ teaspoon sea salt

½ teaspoon dried oregano

½ teaspoon dried basil

1 teaspoon ground turmeric

1 garlic clove, chopped

Place the oil, water, vinegar, salt, oregano, basil, turmeric, and garlic in a blender and blend until smooth.

LEFTOVER TIP: **This sauce stays fresh for 1 week in the refrigerator. You may need to reblend or whisk it to combine before serving.**

Per Serving: Calories: 163; Fat: 18g; Carbohydrates: 1g; Fiber: 0g; Protein: 0g; Sodium: 198mg

Salmon Hummus Wrap

30 minutes or less, 5-ingredient, Dairy-free, No-cook, Nut-free
SERVES 4 | **PREP TIME:** 10 minutes

Lunch does not need to be complicated; this recipe is a perfect example of that! It's super easy and super delicious. Try it and see. Creamy hummus mixed with fresh, crunchy celery and flaky tuna makes a delicious filling for these healthy, easy lunch wraps.

2 (5-ounce) cans wild salmon, drained (see Substitution Tip)

½ cup Roasted Garlic Hummus (page 87)

4 celery stalks, chopped

4 (10-inch) whole-wheat tortillas

8 romaine lettuce leaves

1. In a medium bowl, mix the salmon with the hummus and celery.

2. Place a quarter of the mixture on each wrap. Top each with 2 romaine lettuce leaves and roll up to make the wrap.

> SUBSTITUTION TIP: **Replace the salmon with canned (or leftover) chicken or tuna to change the protein source in these easy wraps.**

Per Serving (with Roasted Garlic Hummus)**:** Calories: 327; Fat: 14g; Carbohydrates: 26g; Fiber: 8g; Protein: 26g; Sodium: 694mg

Roasted Garlic Hummus

Dairy-free, Gluten-free, Nut-free, Vegan
SERVES 8 | **PREP TIME:** 20 minutes | **COOK TIME:** 45 minutes

Raw garlic has a harsh flavor, but roasted garlic has a mild butteriness that adds an unbeatable richness to your hummus. Tahini, also known as sesame seed butter, can be found near the peanut butter in the grocery store.

1 large head garlic

1 teaspoon avocado oil

2 (15-ounce) cans chickpeas, drained and rinsed (see Substitution Tip)

¾ cup warm water

¼ cup tahini

¼ cup extra-virgin olive oil

Juice of 1 lemon (¼ cup)

½ teaspoon sea salt

1. Preheat the oven to 400°F.

2. Cut off the top of the garlic head so the cloves are exposed. It's okay if some cloves detach from the rest of the head. Drizzle the top with the avocado oil. Tightly wrap the garlic head and any cloves that might have fallen off in foil and roast for 45 minutes, until the garlic is fork-tender.

3. Allow the garlic to cool completely; then squeeze out the cloves from their wrapping and put them in the food processor. Add the chickpeas, water, tahini, olive oil, lemon juice, and salt. Process until smooth and creamy.

4. Taste and adjust the salt as needed.

> **SUBSTITUTION TIP: Out of chickpeas? Use white beans instead for a slightly different flavor.**
>
> **LEFTOVER TIP: The hummus will keep for up to 1 week in the refrigerator or 3 months in the freezer.**

Per Serving: Calories: 256; Fat: 15g; Carbohydrates: 25g; Fiber: 7g; Protein: 9g; Sodium: 163mg

Shepherd's Pie Skillet

Gluten-free, Nut-free
SERVES 4 | **PREP TIME:** 10 minutes | **COOK TIME:** 40 minutes

My husband loves shepherd's pie and has been asking me to make it for him for years. I always hesitate, though, because it can get a little too involved and requires baking in the oven for a long time. That's why for this version of shepherd's pie, I lightened it up with steak instead of ground beef and made it on the stovetop so you don't have to heat up your oven!

- 2 russet potatoes, chopped into ½-inch cubes
- 1 head cauliflower, cut into florets
- 3 tablespoons salted butter, divided
- ½ teaspoon garlic powder
- ½ teaspoon sea salt
- ½ teaspoon freshly ground black pepper
- ¼ cup sour cream
- 3 teaspoons avocado oil, divided
- 1 pound flank steak, cut into small cubes (see Substitution Tip)
- 1 yellow onion, diced
- 4 garlic cloves, minced
- 12 ounces carrots, diced
- 2 tablespoons all-purpose flour or cornstarch
- 2 cups beef broth

1. Place the potatoes in a large pot. Cover them with water, bring to a boil over high heat, and boil until tender, 12 to 15 minutes.

2. While the potatoes are boiling, in another large pot, boil or steam the cauliflower for 4 to 6 minutes until it's fork-tender.

3. Drain the potatoes and put them back in the pot. When the cauliflower is done, drain it and add it to the pot with the potatoes. Using a hand-held electric mixer or a potato masher, mash the potatoes and cauliflower. Then whip in 2 tablespoons of butter and the garlic powder, salt, pepper, and sour cream. Cover the pot and set aside.

4. In a large nonstick skillet over medium heat, add 1 teaspoon of avocado oil and the steak. Cook the steak, stirring frequently, for 3 to 5 minutes or until it's cooked the way you like it. Remove the steak from the pan and set aside.

5. Pour the remaining 2 teaspoons of avocado oil into the same pan; then add the onion and minced garlic. Sauté until the onion is translucent and tender, 2 to 3 minutes. Add the carrots and cook for 7 to 8 minutes, stirring frequently, until they're softened. Add the remaining 1 tablespoon of butter to the pan. When it's melted, stir in the flour.

6. Add the beef broth and simmer until the mixture is thickened, 5 to 8 minutes. Stir the steak back into the pan and just heat through. Turn off the heat. Spread the mashed potato mixture on top, leaving a 1-inch gap around the edges.

7. Serve right from the skillet, spooning it out into four servings at the table.

SUBSTITUTION TIP: You can substitute 90 percent lean ground beef for the steak. To lighten up the recipe even more, you could use 93 percent lean ground turkey.

Per Serving: Calories: 586; Fat: 32g; Carbohydrates: 44g; Fiber: 9g; Protein: 32g; Sodium: 786mg

Farmers' Market Omelets

30 minutes or less, Dairy-free, Gluten-free, Nut-free, Vegetarian
SERVES 4 | **PREP TIME:** 10 minutes | **COOK TIME:** 10 minutes

These savory, cheesy omelets are packed with the bounty of the farmers' market, including zucchini, bell pepper, onion, and garlic. The great thing about this recipe is that you can use whatever vegetables are in season to make a delicious seasonal and local breakfast.

1 tablespoon avocado oil

½ **red onion, diced**

4 **garlic cloves, minced**

1 **red bell pepper, seeded and diced**

1 **zucchini, diced**

10 **asparagus spears, chopped into ½-inch pieces**

¼ **teaspoon sea salt**

¼ **teaspoon freshly ground black pepper**

8 **eggs, divided**

1 **cup liquid 100 percent egg whites, divided**

2 **teaspoons salted butter, divided**

½ **cup shredded Gruyère cheese, divided**

4 **cups strawberries**

1. In a large nonstick skillet over medium heat, combine the oil, onion, and garlic. Sauté for 2 to 3 minutes, until the onion is translucent and tender. Add the bell pepper, zucchini, and asparagus to the pan and sauté until softened. Sprinkle with the salt and pepper. Remove the veggies from the skillet and set aside.

2. In a small bowl, whisk together 2 eggs and ¼ cup of egg whites.

3. To the same skillet, add ½ teaspoon of butter and the egg mixture. Tilt the pan to cover the bottom with the eggs. Spoon one-quarter of the veggies in the center of the eggs and top with 2 tablespoons of cheese.

4. When the eggs are almost set, fold two edges over the veggies to make an omelet. Remove from the heat and serve. Repeat three times more to make a total of four omelets.

5. Serve with a side of 1 cup of strawberries per person.

LEFTOVER TIP: **Slightly undercook the omelets you know you will be keeping TO EAT ANOTHER DAY.** That way, when you reheat them, they will be perfect!

Per Serving: Calories: 368; Fat: 20g; Carbohydrates: 21g; Fiber: 6g; Protein: 27g; Sodium: 495mg

Fried Cauliflower Rice

30 minutes or less, Dairy-free, Gluten-free, Nut-free, Vegetarian
SERVES 4 | **PREP TIME:** 10 minutes | **COOK TIME:** 20 minutes

Are you craving a big bowl of salty, savory fried rice? This version uses cauliflower rice instead of white rice and sneaks in more veggies. Be sure to try the oyster or fish sauce, both of which are found in the Asian foods aisle and add a deep, rich flavor to the dish.

3 tablespoons plus 1 teaspoon sesame oil, divided

6 eggs, beaten

Sea salt

Freshly ground black pepper

1 bag (24 ounces) frozen cauliflower rice

2 large carrots, cubed (about 1 cup)

½ white onion, chopped

2 garlic cloves, minced

2½ cups frozen shelled edamame

2 scallions, chopped

½ cup coconut aminos or soy sauce

1 tablespoon oyster sauce or fish sauce (optional)

1. Heat 1 teaspoon of sesame oil in a large skillet over medium heat; then add the eggs and scramble them. Season with salt and pepper and remove the eggs from the skillet.

2. In another large skillet, combine 1 tablespoon of sesame oil and the cauliflower rice and cook until it's defrosted and slightly browned on one side, about 8 minutes. Don't overcook and let it get mushy. Remove from the heat and set aside.

3. In another large skillet, combine the carrots, onion, garlic, and edamame with 1 tablespoon of sesame oil and cook over medium heat until the carrots are fork-tender but still firm, about 10 minutes. Stir in the remaining 1 tablespoon of sesame oil.

4. Add the cauliflower rice and scrambled eggs to the vegetables. Then stir in the chopped scallions. Pour the soy sauce and oyster sauce (if using) over everything, mix well, and season with more salt and pepper. Serve immediately.

> PERFECTLY HEALTHY: **Traditional stir-fry is high in fat, but swapping in cauliflower rice keeps the calorie count under control for weight loss.**

Per Serving: Calories: 388; Fat: 22g; Carbohydrates: 24g; Fiber: 8g; Protein: 24g; Sodium: 1,049mg

Vanilla Latte Overnight Oats

Dairy-free, Gluten-free, No-cook, Vegetarian
SERVES 2 | **PREP TIME:** 5 minutes | **CHILL TIME:** 4 hours

I'm a hard-core coffee lover. I love the flavor, I love the energy—and now I love it in oats. These oats, which have a powerful energy boost with a splash of cold brew and taste like your favorite vanilla latte, might be the best oats I've ever tasted.

1 cup rolled oats, divided

1 cup whole milk, divided

½ cup cold brew coffee, divided
(see Substitution Tip)

½ cup vanilla protein powder, divided
(see Substitution Tip)

2 tablespoons almond butter, divided

2 tablespoons chia seeds, divided

1 tablespoon maple syrup, divided

½ teaspoon vanilla extract, divided

1. Divide the oats, milk, coffee, protein powder, almond butter, chia seeds, maple syrup, and vanilla equally between two resealable containers, such as large mason jars. Mix the contents of each container well and place them in the refrigerator for a minimum of 4 hours or up to 5 days.

2. Enjoy hot or cold. To heat, microwave for 1 to 2 minutes.

> SUBSTITUTION TIP: **If you prefer a mocha flavor, use chocolate protein powder instead of vanilla protein powder. If you don't love caffeine, you can make this with decaf cold brew. If you don't drink coffee, try regular or decaffeinated cold chai tea instead.**

Per Serving: Calories: 419; Fat: 18g; Carbohydrates: 45g; Fiber: 10g; Protein: 24g; Sodium: 89mg

Sweet and Spicy Shrimp, Quinoa, and Asparagus

Dairy-free, Gluten-free, Nut-free
SERVES 4 | **PREP TIME:** 10 minutes | **COOK TIME:** 35 minutes

Fresh shrimp tossed with sweet and spicy seasonings, lemony asparagus, and hearty quinoa come together to make a hearty weeknight meal. I love simple dishes like this that combine a healthy protein, a complex carb, and plenty of veggies in one meal. You could easily batch-cook this meal and freeze it for a future week when you aren't following the 30-day program. It should keep for about 3 months in the freezer.

½ **cup uncooked quinoa** (see Substitution Tip)

1 **cup water**

2 **tablespoons avocado oil, divided**

1 **garlic clove, minced**

4 **cups asparagus, cut into 1-inch pieces**

¼ **teaspoon sea salt**

1 **tablespoon freshly squeezed lemon juice**

1 **tablespoon maple syrup**

⅛ **teaspoon cayenne pepper**

½ **teaspoon smoked paprika**

1 **pound raw medium peeled and deveined shrimp (21 to 30)**

1. Combine the quinoa and water in a small pot and bring to a boil over high heat. Turn the heat down to medium-low, cover the pot, and simmer for 12 to 15 minutes, until all the liquid is absorbed and the quinoa is fluffy. Set aside with the pot covered.

2. In a large skillet, heat 1 tablespoon of oil. Add the garlic and sauté on medium-high heat for 1 to 2 minutes, until it's translucent and tender. Add the asparagus and salt and cover the pan. Cook for 10 minutes; then add the lemon juice and stir to combine. Remove the asparagus from the pan and set aside.

3. In a small bowl, mix the maple syrup, remaining 1 tablespoon of oil, the cayenne, and the paprika. Put the mixture in the pan from step 2; then add the shrimp. Cook the shrimp for 3 to 5 minutes on each side, making sure to coat the shrimp with the sauce. Add the asparagus back to the pan and stir just to combine.

continued ▶

Sweet and Spicy Shrimp, Quinoa, and Asparagus *continued*

4. Serve immediately. A serving is one-quarter of the shrimp and asparagus mixture served over one-quarter of the quinoa.

SUBSTITUTION TIP: Feel free to get creative with your grains. Quinoa is a delicious choice, but you could also use whole-wheat orzo, brown rice, or any other hearty whole grain.

Per Serving: Calories: 183; Fat: 9g; Carbohydrates: 23g; Fiber: 4g; Protein: 6g; Sodium: 153mg

Enchilada-Stuffed Zucchini Boats

30 minutes or less, Gluten-free, Nut-free, Vegetarian
SERVES 4 | **PREP TIME:** 10 minutes | **COOK TIME:** 20 minutes

Spicy, flavorful enchilada filling is stuffed into gently roasted zucchini boats for a lighter twist on this delicious classic food.

Nonstick cooking spray

4 medium zucchini (see Substitution Tip)

1 tablespoon avocado oil

2 garlic cloves, minced

1 yellow onion, chopped

1 pound 93 percent lean ground turkey

2 cups enchilada sauce

1 (15-ounce) can whole tomatoes, drained

½ cup shredded Cheddar cheese, divided

1. Preheat the oven to 375°F. Line a large baking sheet with aluminum foil and spray with nonstick cooking spray.

2. Cut the zucchini in half lengthwise, scoop out the seeds, and place the zucchini boats cut-side down on the baking sheet. Roast for 15 minutes.

3. While the zucchini is cooking, in a large nonstick skillet over medium heat, heat the avocado oil, garlic, and onion and sauté for 1 to 2 minutes, until the garlic is fragrant. Add the ground turkey to the pan and cook thoroughly until no pink remains, about 10 minutes. Add the enchilada sauce and tomatoes and let simmer for 5 minutes, or until the water evaporates and the sauce thickens. Use a wooden spoon to break up the tomatoes as they cook.

4. Fill each zucchini half with the turkey meat mixture, top each with 1 tablespoon of shredded cheese, and serve immediately.

SUBSTITUTION TIP: **In the winter, try substituting delicata squash for a fun twist on this recipe. You'll roast the delicata squash for 25 minutes in step 2.**

Per Serving: Calories: 359; Fat: 20g; Carbohydrates: 19g; Fiber: 3g; Protein: 29g; Sodium: 959mg

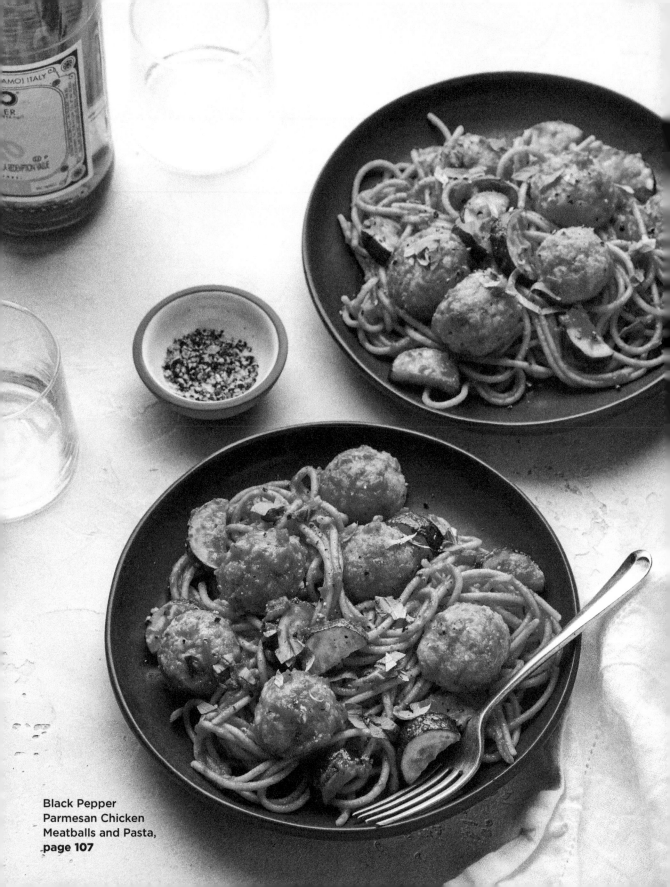

Black Pepper
Parmesan Chicken
Meatballs and Pasta,
page 107

CHAPTER 6

Meal Plan for Days 15 to 21

THIS IS THE THIRD WEEK IN THE PLAN, AND BY NOW YOU SHOULD REALLY BE seeing some awesome success. If you aren't, ask yourself if you are sticking to the plan or veering off it. If you haven't been counting calories, now might be the time to start to help you figure out where you can make more progress. (See chapter 2 for details about how to figure out how many daily calories you need.) Week 3 is where many people fall of the wagon, but *not* you—you're here to see it through. If you can, you must, so keep going!

Your Workouts

Here is a blank chart to plan your workouts for the week based on what you learned in chapter 2.

SUNDAY	MONDAY	TUESDAY	WEDNESDAY	THURSDAY	FRIDAY	SATURDAY

Similar to last week, you should be building up your workouts so that this week you can lift a heavier dumbbell, go a little faster, and see real improvements from week 1. Plan it out in the preceding chart. Enjoy your success. The best part of working out is making progress. Here's a sample chart of where you may be this week.

SUNDAY	MONDAY	TUESDAY	WEDNESDAY	THURSDAY	FRIDAY	SATURDAY
LISS cardio: 30 minutes Stretching or foam rolling: 10 minutes	Full-body strength training: 30 minutes Stretching or foam rolling: 10 minutes	Rest/active recovery: walk, stretch, or light yoga	Full-body strength training: 30 minutes Optional stretching or foam rolling: 10 minutes	HIIT cardio: 20 minutes	Strength and cardio: 30–45 minutes Stretching or foam rolling: 10 minutes	Rest/active recovery: walk, stretch, or light yoga

Your Habit Tracker

Use this chart to help keep yourself accountable for your SMART goals by breaking your big goals into smaller ones.

HABIT	SUN	M	T	W	TH	F	SAT

Meal Plan

WEEK 2	SUN (Daily Calories: 1,676)	M (Daily calories: 1,538)	T (Daily calories: 1,809)	W (Daily calories: 1,647)	TH (Daily calories: 1,505)	F (Daily calories: 1,548)	SAT (Daily calories: 1,606)
Breakfast	Chocolate Power Waffles (page 115)	Protein-Packed Cinnamon French Toast (page 103)	Protein-Packed Coconut Chocolate Steel-Cut Oats (page 105)	Protein-Packed Cinnamon French Toast (leftovers)	Protein-Packed Coconut Chocolate Steel-Cut Oats (leftovers)	Caramelized Banana Power Toast (2 servings) (page 110)	Breakfast Power Bowls (page 111)
Lunch	Chopped Greek Rainbow Salad (page 116)	Sweet and Spicy Shrimp, Quinoa, and Asparagus (leftovers from week 2)	Veggie Black Bean Quesadillas (page 106)	Veggie Black Bean Quesadillas (leftovers)	Lemon Rosemary Shrimp and Orzo Salad (leftovers)	Black Pepper Parmesan Chicken Meatballs and Pasta (leftovers)	Open-Face Caprese Tuna Melts (page 112)
Dinner	Chimichurri Salmon with Roasted Turmeric Cauliflower (leftovers)	Enchilada-Stuffed Zucchini Boats (leftovers from week 2)	Black Pepper Parmesan Chicken Meatballs and Pasta (page 107)	Lemon Rosemary Shrimp and Orzo Salad (page 108)	Slow Cooker Barbecue Chicken–Stuffed Sweet Potatoes (page 109)	Slow Cooker Barbecue Chicken–Stuffed Sweet Potatoes (leftovers)	Chimichurri Salmon with Roasted Turmeric Cauliflower (page 113)
Dessert	Chocolate Chip Edible Cookie Dough (leftovers)	Chocolate Chip Edible Cookie Dough (page 104)	Chocolate Chip Edible Cookie Dough (leftovers)	Chocolate Chip Edible Cookie Dough (leftovers)	Chocolate Chip Edible Cookie Dough (leftovers)	Chocolate Chip Edible Cookie Dough (leftovers)	Chocolate Chip Edible Cookie Dough (leftovers)

Shopping List

Here is your shopping list for the week. Make sure to check out the recipes before heading to the store. If you choose to make substitutions in your recipes, you'll need to update the shopping list. Check your pantry to make sure you don't buy double of any ingredients, especially spices, that you might already have on hand.

Fresh Produce

→ Avocado (1)
→ Banana (1)
→ Basil leaves (1 bunch)
→ Berries, mixed (4 cups)
→ Cauliflower (2 heads)
→ Celery (1 bunch)
→ Cilantro, fresh (1 bunch)
→ Garlic (1 head)
→ Grapes (4 cups)
→ Lemons (4)

→ Lime (1), if making Fresh Homemade Salsa (page 62)
→ Onion, red (1)
→ Onion, white (1), if making Fresh Homemade Salsa (page 62)
→ Parsley, fresh (1 bunch)
→ Peppers, bell, red (2), orange (1), yellow (1)

→ Scallion (1 bunch)
→ Snap peas (4 cups)
→ Spinach, baby (2 cups)
→ Squash, yellow (1)
→ Sweet potatoes (4)
→ Tomatoes, Roma (2, or 8 if making Fresh Homemade Salsa [page 62])
→ Zucchini (3)

Frozen

→ Edamame, shelled, frozen, 1 (14-ounce) bag

Pantry

→ Almond butter, creamy
→ Almonds, unsalted slivered
→ Artichoke hearts, 1 (12-ounce) jar
→ Baking powder
→ Barbecue sauce, low sugar
→ Basil, dried
→ Beans, black, 1 (15-ounce) can
→ Bread crumbs

→ Bread, whole-grain (2 loaves)
→ Cashew butter
→ Cherries, dried
→ Chicken broth, organic, 1 (16-ounce) carton
→ Chickpeas, 2 (15-ounce) cans
→ Chocolate chips, mini
→ Cinnamon

→ Cocoa powder, unsweetened
→ Coconut extract (optional)
→ Coconut flakes, unsweetened
→ Coconut milk, 1 (15-ounce) can
→ Cumin
→ Dates, Medjool (4)
→ Dill, dried
→ Flour, almond (½ cup)

- → Flour, oat (½ cup)
- → Flour, whole-wheat pastry
- → Garlic powder
- → Hemp seeds
- → Honey
- → Italian seasoning
- → Maple syrup
- → Marinara sauce, 1 (16-ounce) jar
- → Mayonnaise, avocado oil
- → Nonstick cooking spray
- → Oats, quick-cooking steel-cut
- → Oil, avocado
- → Oil, coconut
- → Oil, extra-virgin olive
- → Olives, green, 1 (8-ounce) jar
- → Oregano, dried
- → Orzo, whole-wheat, 1 (8-ounce) package
- → Penne, whole-wheat, 1 (8-ounce) package
- → Pepper, black
- → Protein power, chocolate
- → Rosemary, dried
- → Salt, garlic
- → Salt, sea
- → Stevia drops
- → Sugar, coconut
- → Tortillas, whole-wheat, 4 (10-inch)
- → Tuna, water-packed, 2 (5-ounce) cans
- → Turmeric, ground
- → Vanilla extract
- → Vinegar, red wine

Refrigerated

- → Butter, salted (1 stick)
- → Cheese, Gruyère, cubed, or feta crumbles (4 ounces)
- → Cheese, Mexican blend or pepper Jack, shredded, 1 (8-ounce) bag
- → Cheese, mozzarella (4 ounces)
- → Cheese, Parmesan, grated, 1 (5-ounce) container
- → Chicken breast, boneless, skinless (1½ pounds)
- → Chicken, ground, extra-lean (1 pound)
- → Cottage cheese, whole-milk (32 ounces)
- → Egg whites, liquid, 1 (16-ounce) carton
- → Eggs (8)
- → Milk, unsweetened almond (½ pint)
- → Salmon, 4 (6-ounce) fillets
- → Shrimp, medium (21 to 30), peeled and deveined (1 pound)

Protein-Packed Cinnamon French Toast

Dairy-free, Nut-free, Vegetarian
SERVES 4 | **PREP TIME:** 5 minutes | **COOK TIME:** 35 minutes

After the first time I made this, my whole family became *obsessed* with eating it. I now have to keep batches of this French toast in the freezer at all times or I'll be sure to hear about it. I can also navigate whining requests to go out to breakfast with the simple phrase "There is French toast in the freezer." The whiners are gone, and I'm back to enjoying my Sunday morning. This French toast is light and fluffy on the inside, crispy on the outside, and full of cinnamon maple flavor.

4 eggs

½ cup egg whites

2 teaspoons vanilla extract

2 teaspoons cinnamon

Nonstick cooking spray or avocado oil

8 slices whole-grain bread

4 cups mixed berries

4 tablespoons maple syrup

1. In a medium bowl, whisk together the eggs, egg whites, vanilla, and cinnamon.

2. Preheat a large skillet or griddle pan over medium heat and grease with nonstick cooking spray.

3. Dredge 1 slice of bread in the egg mixture and add it to the skillet. Cook for 2 to 4 minutes, until the toast is lightly browned on the bottom; then flip and cook for 2 to 4 minutes on the other side. Repeat with the remaining bread.

4. Serve with the mixed berries and maple syrup. One serving is 2 slices of French toast, 1 cup of berries, and 1 tablespoon of syrup.

> LEFTOVER TIP: **Store the French toast and toppings separately in the refrigerator for up to 3 days. (French toast may be frozen for up to 3 months.) Reheat in the toaster oven or on a hot skillet.**

Per Serving: Calories: 461; Fat: 20g; Carbohydrates: 56g; Fiber: 8g; Protein: 16g; Sodium: 381mg

Chocolate Chip Edible Cookie Dough

30 minutes or less, Gluten-free, No-cook, One pot, Vegan
SERVES 8 | **PREP TIME:** 10 minutes

Stick your spoon in the cookie dough jar and feel good about it! Every bite is full of chunky cookie dough and chocolate chips. This divine dessert is intended to be eaten raw and will not actually bake into cookies.

1 (15-ounce) can chickpeas, drained and rinsed (see Substitution Tip)

½ cup oat flour

½ cup cashew butter (see Substitution Tip)

⅓ cup maple syrup

3 or 4 Medjool dates, pitted

1 teaspoon vanilla extract

2 tablespoons to ½ cup almond milk

3 tablespoons mini chocolate chips

1. Put the chickpeas, oat flour, cashew butter, maple syrup, dates, and vanilla in a food processor and process until smooth. If the dough is too chunky, add the almond milk 1 tablespoon at a time.

2. When you have the texture you want, scrape the mixture into a bowl and stir in the chocolate chips.

3. Roll into balls, or just eat with a spoon!

SUBSTITUTION TIP: **You can also use white beans in this recipe. Substitute peanut butter for cashew butter to make peanut butter cookie dough.**

LEFTOVER TIP: **This cookie dough will stay fresh in the refrigerator for 5 to 7 days.**

Per Serving: Calories: 274; Fat: 12g; Carbohydrates: 35g; Fiber: 5g; Protein: 7g; Sodium: 52mg

Protein-Packed Coconut Chocolate Steel-Cut Oats

30 minutes or less, Dairy-free, Gluten-free, Nut-free, One pot, Vegan
SERVES 4 | **PREP TIME:** 5 minutes | **COOK TIME:** 15 minutes

This steaming bowl of coconut chocolate creamy steel-cut oats includes bits of crunchy dried coconut in every bite. It tastes like a Mounds candy bar—and if you want nuts, add crunchy almonds on top.

3 cups water

1 cup quick-cooking steel-cut oats (see Substitution Tip)

1 cup canned coconut milk

1 cup chocolate protein powder

2 tablespoons unsweetened cocoa powder

½ teaspoon coconut extract (optional)

4 tablespoons unsweetened dried coconut flakes, divided

1. In a medium pot over high heat, bring the water to a boil and add the oats. Lower the heat and simmer for 5 to 7 minutes, until the liquid is mostly or completely absorbed. Remove the oats from the heat, cover the pot, and let sit for 5 minutes to thicken.

2. Stir in the coconut milk, protein powder, cocoa powder, and coconut extract (if using) until smooth.

3. Divide among four bowls. Top each serving with 1 tablespoon of coconut flakes.

> SUBSTITUTION TIP: **You can use thick-cut rolled oats, but you'll need 2 cups instead of 1 cup.**

Per Serving: Calories: 414; Fat: 19g; Carbohydrates: 37g; Fiber: 6g; Protein: 25g; Sodium: 59mg

Veggie Black Bean Quesadillas

30 minutes or less, Gluten-free, Nut-free, Vegetarian
SERVES 4 | **PREP TIME:** 10 minutes | **COOK TIME:** 10 minutes

A quesadilla is a kind of taco sandwich—tortillas filled with something delicious and then usually heated to melt the cheese inside and make them crispy on the outside. Mouthwatering, fresh, grilled veggies are combined with your favorite cheese in this delightfully crispy version.

- ¼ **red onion, cut into thin strips**
- 1 **red bell pepper, seeded and cut into thin strips**
- 1 **zucchini, cut into thin strips**
- 1 **yellow squash, cut into thin strips**
- 1 **tablespoon avocado oil**
- ⅛ **teaspoon cumin**
- ½ **teaspoon garlic powder**
- ¼ **teaspoon sea salt**
- 1 **cup black beans, divided**
- 1 **cup shredded Mexican cheese blend or pepper Jack, divided**
- 4 **(10-inch) whole-wheat tortillas**
- **Fresh Homemade Salsa, for garnish** (optional; page 62)

1. Preheat a grill pan on the stovetop over medium heat.

2. In a large bowl, toss the onion, bell pepper, zucchini, and yellow squash with the oil, cumin, garlic, and salt.

3. Grill the vegetables over high heat until grill marks form and the veggies are slightly tender, about 6 to 8 minutes; then remove them from the pan.

4. Add one-quarter of the veggie mixture, ¼ cup of black beans, and ¼ cup of cheese to each tortilla. Fold the tortillas in half to make quesadillas. Place the quesadillas on the same grill pan on medium heat to brown the tortillas and melt the cheese.

5. Serve with Fresh Homemade Salsa on the side (if using).

SUBSTITUTION TIP: **Try using mozzarella and feta cheeses mixed with a little Italian seasoning for a Mediterranean vibe.**

COOKING TIP: **If you don't have a grill pan, just use a large nonstick skillet. You won't get grill marks, but it will still be delicious.**

Per Serving (without the optional Fresh Homemade Salsa)**:** Calories: 516; Fat: 30g; Carbohydrates: 36g; Fiber: 10g; Protein: 27g; Sodium: 665mg

Black Pepper Parmesan Chicken Meatballs and Pasta

Nut-free

SERVES 4 | **PREP TIME:** 10 minutes | **COOK TIME:** 25 minutes

I like these juicy, flavorful meatballs as a protein snack during the day. Toss with marinara, roasted zucchini slices, and pasta for a full meal.

Nonstick cooking spray

1 pound extra-lean ground chicken

½ cup grated Parmesan cheese

½ cup bread crumbs

2 eggs

½ teaspoon sea salt

½ teaspoon freshly ground black pepper

2 large zucchini

1 tablespoon avocado oil

1 teaspoon Italian seasoning

½ teaspoon garlic salt

8 ounces whole-wheat penne or spaghetti pasta

2 cups marinara sauce

½ cup chopped fresh basil, for garnish

1. Preheat the oven to 375°F. Set one rack in the top of the oven and one rack in the bottom. Line two large baking sheets with aluminum foil and grease them with nonstick cooking spray.

2. In a medium bowl, mix the chicken with the Parmesan, bread crumbs, eggs, salt, and pepper. Form into 24 balls and place them on one of the prepared baking sheets. Bake on the top rack for 20 to 25 minutes, until cooked through.

3. Meanwhile, cut the zucchini in half lengthwise and then into ½-inch half-moons. Spread them on the other baking sheet and toss with the avocado oil, Italian seasoning, and garlic salt. Roast for 20 minutes.

4. While the meatballs and zucchini are cooking, cook the pasta according to the directions on the package.

5. In a large bowl, toss the pasta with the marinara sauce and the zucchini. Divide into four bowls and top each with 6 meatballs. Garnish with fresh basil and serve.

Per Serving: Calories: 571; Fat: 23g; Carbohydrates: 55g; Fiber: 6g; Protein: 37g; Sodium: 636mg

Lemon Rosemary Shrimp and Orzo Salad

30 minutes or less, Dairy-free, Nut-free
SERVES 4 | **PREP TIME:** 10 minutes | **COOK TIME:** 20 minutes

If you've never tried orzo before, step out of your comfort zone and do it. It's easy to find at the supermarket, and it's not annoying to cook—my two biggest barriers to entry when looking at new ingredients. I promise you that the chewy texture of whole-wheat orzo will make all the difference in this cold salad recipe. Lemony shrimp, juicy marinated artichokes, and crispy sugar snap peas mix together for a refreshing and filling mix-it-all-up salad.

8 ounces whole-wheat orzo

1 tablespoon avocado oil

1 pound raw medium peeled and deveined shrimp (21 to 30) (see Substitution Tip)

4 cups sugar snap peas (about 20 ounces), trimmed

½ teaspoon sea salt, plus a sprinkle

¼ teaspoon freshly ground black pepper, plus a sprinkle

1 cup green olives, pitted

1 (12-ounce jar) marinated artichokes, drained and quartered

¼ cup lemon juice

1 teaspoon dried rosemary

1. Bring a medium pot of water to a boil over high heat, add the orzo, and cook for 7 to 9 minutes, until al dente. Drain and set aside.

2. Heat the oil in a large skillet over medium heat. Add the shrimp and sugar snap peas. Sprinkle with salt and pepper. Cook the shrimp for 3 to 5 minutes on each side, stirring the snap peas frequently, until the shrimp is pink and hot throughout. Transfer the shrimp and peas to a large serving bowl.

3. Add the orzo, olives, artichokes, and lemon juice. Stir in the rosemary and a sprinkle of salt and pepper and serve immediately.

SUBSTITUTION TIP: **Replace the shrimp with diced chicken for a heartier version of this meal.**

Per Serving: Calories: 396; Fat: 6g; Carbohydrates: 57g; Fiber: 8g; Protein: 33g; Sodium: 730mg

Slow Cooker Barbecue Chicken–Stuffed Sweet Potatoes

5-ingredient, Dairy-free, Gluten-free, Nut-free
SERVES 4 | **PREP TIME:** 10 minutes | **COOK TIME:** 4 hours on high or 6 hours on low

You may have doubts about stuffing barbecue chicken into a sweet potato. My family did. But then they were blown away with how easy and delicious the meal was. These make for a flavorful and filling dinner!

1½ pounds boneless, skinless chicken breasts (see Cooking Tip)

2 cups chicken broth

Nonstick cooking spray or avocado oil

4 sweet potatoes

½ cup low-sugar barbecue sauce (see Perfectly Healthy note)

2 cups baby spinach

1. Put the chicken and broth in a slow cooker and cook on high for 4 hours or on low for 6 hours.

2. When the chicken has 1 hour left, preheat the oven to 400°F. Line a medium baking sheet with aluminum foil and grease it with nonstick cooking spray.

3. Cut a few slits in the sweet potatoes and place them on the baking sheet. Roast for 1 hour. They are done when they are fork-tender.

4. When the chicken is done, remove it from the slow cooker. Shred the chicken with two forks and put it in a medium bowl. Toss the chicken with the barbecue sauce.

5. Cut the sweet potatoes lengthwise almost in half, leaving a pocket in the middle, and stuff with spinach and barbecue chicken. Serve immediately.

PERFECTLY HEALTHY: **Choose barbecue sauce with fewer than 25 calories per serving and minimal sugar to keep calories in check.**

COOKING TIP: **A basic slow cooker is less than $30, and it's the best small appliance you could ever have. I use mine at least once a week! However, you can use shredded rotisserie chicken instead.**

Per Serving: Calories: 327; Fat: 5g; Carbohydrates: 27g; Fiber: 4g; Protein: 41g; Sodium: 622mg

Caramelized Banana Power Toast

30 minutes or less, Vegetarian
SERVES 2 | **PREP TIME:** 10 minutes | **COOK TIME:** 10 minutes

Yes, toast can be a healthy breakfast! I hate that bread has been vilified. It's true that most Americans eat way too much bread and white refined carbs in general, but whole-grain bread once a day is good for you; it supplies vitamins, fiber, and protein. This hearty whole-grain toast is smothered with creamy almond butter, nutty hemp seeds, and golden-sweet caramelized bananas.

2 large slices whole-grain bread

2 tablespoons almond butter (see Substitution Tip)

2 tablespoons hemp seeds (see Perfectly Healthy note)

1½ teaspoons salted butter

1½ teaspoons coconut sugar

1 large banana, sliced

1. Toast the 2 slices of bread; then spread each slice with half the almond butter and sprinkle on the hemp seeds.

2. In a small nonstick skillet over medium heat, heat the butter. Add the sugar and banana slices. Sauté for 5 minutes until caramelized. Spoon onto the toast.

SUBSTITUTION TIP: **Swap the almond butter for any other type of nut or seed butter.**

PERFECTLY HEALTHY: **Hemp seeds, also called hemp hearts, are a good source of anti-inflammatory omega-3-rich healthy fats and protein. They make your toast just a bit heartier, plus they add a lovely nutty flavor and chewy texture. Find them in supermarkets and health food stores.**

Per Serving: Calories: 316; Fat: 19g; Carbohydrates: 32g; Fiber: 5g; Protein: 9g; Sodium: 130mg

Breakfast Power Bowls

30 minutes or less, 5-ingredient, Gluten-free, No-cook, Vegetarian
SERVES 4 | **PREP TIME:** 10 minutes

Top creamy whole-milk cottage cheese with fresh, juicy grapes and chopped almonds and drizzle it with honey for a healthy breakfast treat that will keep you feeling full. It's an easy breakfast that's good for you and is delicious.

4 cups whole-milk cottage cheese, divided (see Substitution Tip)

4 cups grapes, halved, divided (see Substitution Tip)

½ cup unsalted slivered almonds, divided (see Substitution Tip)

4 tablespoons honey, divided

Set out four bowls. Add 1 cup of cottage cheese, 1 cup of grapes, 2 tablespoons of chopped almonds, and 1 tablespoon of honey to each bowl. Serve.

SUBSTITUTION TIP: **If you don't like or have cottage cheese, you could also use plain Greek yogurt. Feel free to use the same quantities but vary the types of fruit and nuts for different combinations.**

Per Serving: Calories: 432; Fat: 18g; Carbohydrates: 43g; Fiber: 3g; Protein: 28g; Sodium: 663mg

Open-Face Caprese Tuna Melts

30 minutes or less, Nut-free, Sheet pan
SERVES 4 | **PREP TIME:** 10 minutes | **COOK TIME:** 20 minutes

Get ready for a tuna melt with a twist. A traditional caprese salad is made with sliced fresh mozzarella, tomatoes, and sweet basil seasoned with salt and olive oil. In this more substantial version, tuna salad is piled on top of fresh, juicy tomato slices, topped with mozzarella, and then baked until the cheese is bubbly and slightly golden brown around the edges.

2 (5-ounce) cans tuna packed in water, drained (see Substitution Tip)

1 avocado, smashed

2 celery stalks, chopped

2 tablespoons avocado oil mayonnaise

½ teaspoon Italian seasoning

¼ teaspoon dried dill

⅛ teaspoon sea salt

⅛ teaspoon freshly ground black pepper

8 pieces thin-sliced whole-grain bread

2 Roma tomatoes, sliced

4 ounces shredded mozzarella cheese, divided

4 tablespoons chopped fresh basil, divided, plus more for garnish

1. Preheat the oven to 375°F. Line a large baking sheet with aluminum foil.

2. In a large bowl, mix the tuna, avocado, celery, mayonnaise, Italian seasoning, dill, salt, and pepper.

3. Lay out the bread slices on the prepared baking sheet. Top each with 1 tomato slice, one-eighth of the tuna mixture, ½ ounce of mozzarella, and 1½ teaspoons of fresh basil.

4. Bake for 10 to 20 minutes, until the cheese is hot and bubbly. Garnish with more fresh basil. Serve immediately.

SUBSTITUTION TIP: **You can also use canned chicken or leftover cooked chicken in this recipe for a different protein option.**

Per Serving: Calories: 445; Fat: 23g; Carbohydrates: 33g; Fiber: 7g; Protein: 27g; Sodium: 663mg

Chimichurri Salmon with Roasted Turmeric Cauliflower

30 minutes or less, Dairy-free, Gluten-free, Nut-free
SERVES 4 | **PREP TIME:** 10 minutes | **COOK TIME:** 20 minutes

Seafood is one of the most nutrition-packed protein sources you can eat, especially salmon. Wild-caught salmon and salmon raised in humane farms (as is the practice in most of Europe and the United States) is packed with anti-inflammatory fatty acids that fight chronic disease. Farmed salmon from other areas of the globe should be avoided due to chemical and pollutant contamination. It is also typically lower in omega-3 fatty acids.

FOR THE CAULIFLOWER
Nonstick cooking spray

6 cups cauliflower florets (about 2 medium heads)

1 tablespoon avocado oil

¾ teaspoon ground turmeric

½ teaspoon garlic powder

¼ teaspoon sea salt

FOR THE SALMON
1½ teaspoons sea salt

¼ teaspoon freshly ground black pepper

1 garlic clove

1 bunch parsley, stems removed, leaves chopped

1 cup chopped fresh cilantro

1 scallion, chopped

¼ cup avocado oil

2 tablespoons red wine vinegar

1 tablespoon freshly squeezed lemon juice

4 (6-ounce) salmon fillets (see Substitution Tip)

TO MAKE THE CAULIFLOWER

1. Preheat the oven to 400°F. Set one rack in the top of the oven and one rack in the bottom. Line two baking sheets with aluminum foil and spray with nonstick cooking spray.

2. Add the cauliflower to one of the prepared baking sheets and toss with the avocado oil, turmeric, garlic powder, and salt. (You may need to rub the seasonings in by hand.) Bake on the top rack for 20 minutes, until fork-tender.

continued ▶

Chimichurri Salmon with Roasted Turmeric Cauliflower *continued*

3. In a small bowl, blend the salt, pepper, garlic, parsley, cilantro, scallion, avocado oil, vinegar, and lemon juice.

4. Place the salmon fillets skin-side down on the other prepared baking sheet and spoon 1 or 2 tablespoons of chimichurri sauce over each piece of salmon. Bake on the bottom rack for 15 to 20 minutes, until it's cooked the way you like. Some people like their salmon a little less done than others, but I prefer flaky throughout and an internal temperature of at least 145°F. Serve immediately with the roasted cauliflower.

SUBSTITUTION TIP: **You can substitute cod for the salmon. This lemony sauce pairs well with white fish.**

Per Serving: Calories: 455; Fat: 26g; Carbohydrates: 18g; Fiber: 7g; Protein: 41g; Sodium: 1,069mg

Chocolate Power Waffles

30 minutes or less, Vegetarian
SERVES 4 | **PREP TIME:** 10 minutes | **COOK TIME:** 20 minutes

Chocolate for breakfast, anyone? These power waffles are light and fluffy on the inside, crispy on the outside, and drizzled with a syrup that will have you licking your plate. If you don't have a waffle iron, you can use this batter to make pancakes instead.

Nonstick cooking spray

½ cup almond flour

½ cup whole-wheat pastry flour

2 tablespoons unsweetened cocoa powder

1 teaspoon baking powder

¼ teaspoon sea salt

2 eggs

1 tablespoon maple syrup

1 tablespoon coconut oil

½ cup unsweetened almond milk

5 drops liquid stevia (optional)

¼ cup Almond Butter Syrup (page 80) **or maple syrup**

1. Preheat a four-waffle Belgian waffle iron and spray it with nonstick cooking spray.

2. In a large bowl, whisk together the almond flour, whole-wheat pastry flour, cocoa powder, baking powder, and salt.

3. In another large bowl, whisk together the eggs, maple syrup, coconut oil, milk, and stevia (if using). Add the wet ingredients to the dry and mix until everything is well combined.

4. Pour the mixture into the waffle iron and cook for 5 to 10 minutes, or until the waffle maker says it's ready. Serve each waffle with 1 tablespoon of syrup on top.

COOKING TIP: If you don't have a Belgian waffle iron, you'll have to adjust this recipe and make the waffles in batches. One-quarter of the recipe makes one large Belgian waffle, so adjust according to the size of your waffle iron.

Per Serving (with Almond Butter Syrup)**:** Calories: 319; Fat: 24g; Carbohydrates: 21g; Fiber: 5g; Protein: 10g; Sodium: 328mg

Chopped Greek Rainbow Salad

30 minutes or less, Gluten-free, No-cook, Nut-free, One bowl, Vegetarian
SERVES 4 | **PREP TIME:** 15 minutes

Every color of fruits and veggies has unique health benefits, and that's why it's so important to "eat the rainbow." In this delicious Greek salad, you'll have a beautiful mix of colorful veggies tossed with cheese, olive oil, and herbs for a refreshing, crunchy salad.

- **2 cups shelled frozen edamame**
- **1 orange bell pepper, seeded and chopped**
- **1 yellow bell pepper, seeded and chopped**
- **1 red bell pepper, seeded and chopped**

- **1 (15-ounce) can chickpeas, drained and rinsed**
- **½ cup cubed Gruyère or feta cheese**
- **2 tablespoons extra-virgin olive oil**
- **2 tablespoons fresh lemon juice**

- **½ teaspoon garlic salt**
- **½ teaspoon freshly ground black pepper**
- **½ teaspoon Italian seasoning**
- **½ teaspoon dried basil**
- **½ teaspoon dried oregano**

1. In a microwave-safe dish, microwave the frozen edamame for 3 to 5 minutes, until tender and hot throughout. Let cool slightly in the refrigerator while you make the rest of the salad.

2. In a large mixing bowl, toss the bell peppers, chickpeas, cheese, olive oil, lemon juice, garlic salt, black pepper, Italian seasoning, basil, and oregano. Add the cooled edamame and toss to combine.

3. Divide into four bowls to serve.

LEFTOVER TIP: **This salad is a great make-ahead because it stays fresh for a few days in the refrigerator without getting soggy.**

Per Serving: Calories: 367; Fat: 17g; Carbohydrates: 35g; Fiber: 12g; Protein: 21g; Sodium: 189mg

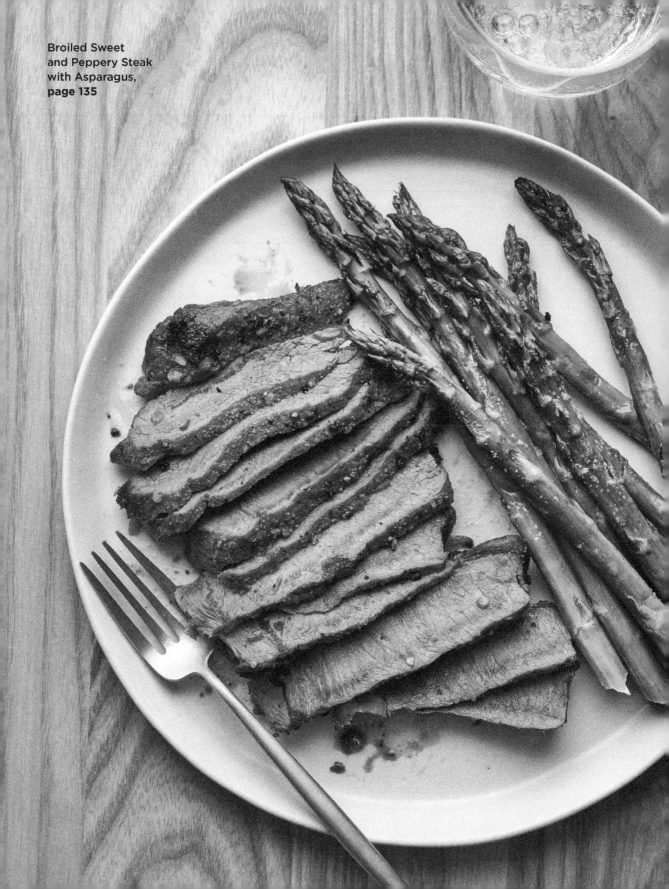

Broiled Sweet
and Peppery Steak
with Asparagus,
page 135

CHAPTER 7

Meal Plan
for Days 22 to 30

IF YOU ARE READING THIS, YOU'VE MADE IT TO THE FINAL WEEK.
Congratulations! This is a *huge* accomplishment. Now, even if you've had
some setbacks in the past few weeks, it's time to finish strong. Remember:
Anyone can start, but it only counts if you finish. And getting to the finish
line is what matters, not whether you've been perfect up until now!

Remember, this first 30 days is just a jump start to the beginning of the
rest of your life on your healthy living journey. At the end of these 30 days,
take out a pen and paper and write down all the things you are proud of:
what you learned, what you did, and how you accomplished it. These things
will be only a drop in the bucket compared to what you'll accomplish going
forward now that you have the tools to make a lasting impact on your health.

Your Workouts

Here is a blank chart to plan your workouts for the week based on what you learned in chapter 2.

SUNDAY	MONDAY	TUESDAY	WEDNESDAY	THURSDAY	FRIDAY	SATURDAY

Your workouts should have been building every single week so that this week you can lift a little more, go a little faster, and see real improvements from week 1. Enjoy it. The best part of working out is making progress. Here's a sample exercise chart for this week.

SUNDAY	MONDAY	TUESDAY	WEDNESDAY	THURSDAY	FRIDAY	SATURDAY
LISS cardio: 30 minutes Stretching or foam rolling: 10 minutes	Full-body strength training: 30 minutes Stretching or foam rolling: 10 minutes	Rest/active recovery: walk, stretch, or light yoga	Full-body strength training: 30 minutes Optional stretching or foam rolling: 10 minutes	HIIT cardio: 20 minutes	Strength and cardio: 30–45 minutes Stretching or foam rolling: 10 minutes	Rest/active recovery: walk, stretch, or light yoga

Your Habit Tracker

Use this chart to help keep yourself accountable for your SMART goals by breaking your big goals into smaller ones.

HABIT	SUN	M	T	W	TH	F	SAT

Meal Plan

WEEK 4	SUN (Daily calories: 1,522)	M (Daily calories: 1,639)	T (Daily calories: 1,525)	W (Daily calories: 1,601)	TH (Daily calories: 1,519)	F (Daily calories: 1,755)	SAT (Daily calories: 1,455)
Breakfast	Orange Dreamsicle Protein Smoothie (2 servings)	Breakfast Power Bowls (leftovers from week 3)	Chocolate Power Waffles (leftovers from week 3)	Spinach, Red Pepper, and Gruyère Egg Bites (page 129)	Sunshine Lentil Breakfast Bowls (page 131)	Sunshine Lentil Breakfast Bowls (leftovers)	Spinach, Red Pepper, and Gruyere Egg Bites (leftovers)
Lunch	Spanakopita Veggie Burgers with Mixed Greens (leftovers)	Open-Face Caprese Tuna Melts (leftovers from week 3)	Chopped Greek Rainbow Salad (leftovers from week 3)	Soy-Ginger Pork Lettuce Wraps (page 130)	Soy-Ginger Pork Lettuce Wraps (leftovers)	Strawberry Basil Chicken Salad with Baked Goat Cheese (page 133)	Broiled Sweet and Peppery Steak with Asparagus (leftovers)
Dinner	Green Chile Beef Tacos with Cherry Tomato Salad (page 139)	Pesto and Brussels Sprouts Pasta Bake (page 125)	Chicken Fingers and Cheesy Potatoes (page 127)	Pesto and Brussels Sprouts Pasta Bake (leftovers)	Chicken Fingers and Cheesy Potatoes (leftovers)	Broiled Sweet and Peppery Steak with Asparagus (page 135)	Spanakopita Veggie Burgers with Mixed Greens (page 137) (freeze oranges and banana for Orange Dreamsicle Protein Smoothie) (page 138)
Dessert	Skillet Apples and Sunflower Seed Butter (page 126)	Skillet Apples and Sunflower Seed Butter (leftovers)	Skillet Apples and Sunflower Seed Butter (leftovers)	Skillet Apples and Sunflower Seed Butter (leftovers)	Skillet Apples and Sunflower Seed Butter (leftovers)	Skillet Apples and Sunflower Seed Butter (leftovers)	Skillet Apples and Sunflower Seed Butter (leftovers)

	DAY 29 (Daily Calories: 1,808)	DAY 30 (Daily Calories: 1,656)
Breakfast	Black Bean Breakfast Burritos (page 141)	Black Bean Breakfast Burritos (leftovers)
Lunch	Strawberry Basil Chicken Salad with Baked Goat Cheese (leftovers)	Green Chile Beef Tacos with Cherry Tomato Side Salad (leftovers)
Dinner	Vegan Thai-Style Curry (page 142)	Vegan Thai-Style Curry (leftovers)

Shopping List

Here is your shopping list for the week. Make sure to check out the recipes before heading to the store. If you choose to make substitutions in your recipes, you'll need to update the shopping list. Check your pantry to make sure you don't buy double of any ingredients, especially spices, that you might already have on hand.

Fresh Produce

- Apples (4)
- Asparagus (3½ pounds)
- Banana (1)
- Basil, fresh (1 bunch)
- Brussels sprouts (10 ounces)
- Cabbage, green (1 head)
- Cabbage, red (1 head)
- Carrots, shredded (4 ounces)
- Celery (1 bunch)
- Cilantro, fresh (1 bunch), if making Fresh
- Homemade Salsa (page 62)
- Garlic (1 head)
- Lemon (1)
- Lettuce, butter (1 head)
- Lime (1), if making Fresh Homemade Salsa (page 62)
- Mixed greens (12 cups)
- Onion, white (1), if making Fresh Homemade Salsa (page 62)
- Onion, yellow (1)
- Oranges, navel (2)
- Peppers, bell, red (2)
- Pepper, jalapeño (1), if making Fresh Homemade Salsa (page 62)
- Potatoes, russet (4)
- Scallion (1 bunch), if making Fresh Homemade Salsa (page 62)
- Strawberries (2 pints)
- Tomatoes, cherry (2 pints)
- Tomatoes, Roma (6), if making Fresh Homemade Salsa (page 62)

Pantry

- Barbecue sauce, ranch dressing, or honey mustard
- Beans, black, 1 (15-ounce) can
- Bread crumbs, panko
- Bread crumbs, whole-wheat
- Chickpea pasta, 1 (8-ounce) package
- Chiles, green, 1 (4-ounce) can
- Chili powder
- Chinese five-spice powder
- Cinnamon
- Coconut aminos or soy sauce
- Dill, dried
- Flour, almond
- Garlic powder
- Ginger, ground
- Hoisin sauce
- Honey
- Lentils
- Maple syrup

- Nonstick cooking spray
- Nutmeg, ground
- Oil, avocado
- Oil, extra-virgin olive
- Oil, sesame
- Onion flakes
- Onion powder
- Orange extract
- Oregano, dried
- Paprika, smoked
- Peanut butter
- Pepper, black
- Pepper, lemon
- Pesto
- Protein powder, vanilla
- Red pepper flakes
- Rice, brown
- Salad dressing (of your choice)
- Salt, garlic
- Salt, sea
- Sriracha (optional)
- Sugar, coconut
- Sunflower seed butter
- Taco seasoning
- Tahini
- Thai curry sauce. 1 (16-ounce) jar
- Tomatoes, diced, 2 (15-ounce) cans
- Tortillas, 8 (6-inch) corn
- Tortillas, 4 (10-inch) whole-wheat
- Turmeric, ground
- Vanilla extract
- Vinegar, balsamic
- Walnuts, shelled

Frozen
- Brown rice, precooked frozen, 1 (10-ounce) bag (omit if using uncooked rice)
- Spinach, frozen, 2 (10-ounce) packages
- Vegetables, frozen stir-fry mix, 1 (1-pound) bag

Refrigerated
- Beef, 90 percent lean ground (1 pound)
- Butter, salted (1 stick)
- Cheese, Cheddar (7 ounces)
- Cheese, feta, crumbled, 1 (12-ounce) tub
- Cheese, Gruyère, shredded, 1 (6-ounce) package
- Cheese, honey goat, 1 (8-ounce) log
- Cheese, Monterey Jack, shredded, 1 (8-ounce) package
- Cheese, mozzarella, shredded, 1 (8-ounce) package
- Chicken breast (1½ pounds)
- Chicken tenders (1 pound)
- Egg whites, liquid (1 cup)
- Eggs (28)
- Flatiron steaks, 4 (8 ounces)
- Milk, unsweetened almond (1½ cup)
- Pork, lean ground (1 pound)
- Tofu, high-protein or extra-firm (1 pound)

Pesto and Brussels Sprouts Pasta Bake

5-ingredient, Nut-free, Vegetarian
SERVES 4 | **PREP TIME:** 10 minutes | **COOK TIME:** 30 minutes

Who says you can't have comfort food when you're trying to lose weight? This creamy pesto pasta is tossed with Brussels sprouts and topped with a layer of bubbly golden mozzarella cheese for a comfort food that is satisfying and delicious! In a store-bought pesto, I just look for ingredients that I can pronounce. Simple is best!

Nonstick cooking spray

3 cups Brussels sprouts, quartered

1 tablespoon avocado oil

¼ teaspoon sea salt

¼ teaspoon freshly ground black pepper

8 ounces chickpea pasta

½ cup pesto

½ cup shredded mozzarella cheese

1. Preheat the oven to 400°F. Line a baking sheet with aluminum foil and spray with nonstick cooking spray.

2. Spread out the Brussels sprouts on the baking sheet and toss with the avocado oil, salt, and pepper. Roast for 20 minutes or until they're fork-tender.

3. While the Brussels sprouts are roasting, cook the pasta according to the package directions.

4. Preheat the broiler.

5. Transfer the Brussels sprouts and pasta to a 9-by-13-inch baking pan. Toss with the pesto and top with the mozzarella cheese. Broil for 1 to 2 minutes, until the cheese is golden brown and bubbly. Serve.

> PERFECTLY HEALTHY: **Chickpea pasta is made from chickpea flour and is a high-protein, lower-carb, great-tasting alternative to traditional wheat pasta.**

Per Serving: Calories: 450; Fat: 24g; Carbohydrates: 41g; Fiber: 11g; Protein: 24g; Sodium: 505mg

Skillet Apples and Sunflower Seed Butter

30 minutes or less, 5-ingredient, Gluten-free, One pot, Vegetarian
SERVES 8 | **PREP TIME:** 10 minutes | **COOK TIME:** 15 minutes

This is one of my go-to desserts when I need something sweet and a plain piece of fruit is just not going to cut it. Each serving is topped with creamy sunflower seed butter for a healthy dessert. If you have leftovers, reheat the apples before you add the seed or nut butter.

1 tablespoon salted butter

4 apples, chopped

½ teaspoon cinnamon

¼ teaspoon ground nutmeg

4 tablespoons sunflower seed butter, divided
(see Substitution Tip)

1. Melt the butter in a large nonstick skillet over medium heat. Add the apples and sprinkle with cinnamon and nutmeg. Cover the skillet and cook until the apples are tender, about 15 minutes.

2. Top each serving with 1½ teaspoons of sunflower seed butter.

SUBSTITUTION TIP: **Swap the sunflower butter for any other nut or seed butter, such as peanut butter, cashew butter, or almond butter.**

Per Serving: Calories: 110; Fat: 6g; Carbohydrates: 15g; Fiber: 3g; Protein: 2g; Sodium: 1mg

Chicken Fingers and Cheesy Potatoes

30 minutes or less, Sheet pan
SERVES 4 | **PREP TIME:** 10 minutes | **COOK TIME:** 20 minutes

---

You'd think those chicken fingers from your childhood aren't exactly health food, but think again! These chicken tenders are breaded with a combo of whole-wheat bread crumbs, almond flour, and delicious spices and then baked to crispy perfection. Here they're paired with cheesy potato rounds and fresh, crunchy celery for a kid-friendly meal that's all grown up.

FOR THE CHICKEN

Nonstick cooking spray

¼ cup almond flour

¼ cup whole-wheat bread crumbs

1 teaspoon smoked paprika

½ teaspoon garlic powder

½ teaspoon sea salt

¼ teaspoon chili powder

1 egg

1 pound chicken tenders

FOR THE POTATOES

2 russet potatoes (see Substitution Tip)

1 tablespoon avocado oil

1 teaspoon garlic powder

½ teaspoon sea salt

½ teaspoon dried dill

¼ teaspoon onion powder

¼ teaspoon freshly ground black pepper

⅓ cup shredded Cheddar cheese

TO SERVE

4 cups celery sticks

1 cup low-sugar dipping sauce (such as barbecue, ranch, or honey mustard)

TO MAKE THE CHICKEN

1. Preheat the oven to 400°F. Set one rack in the top of the oven and one in the bottom. Line two baking sheets with aluminum foil and spray with nonstick cooking spray.

2. In a medium bowl, mix together the almond flour, bread crumbs, paprika, garlic powder, salt, and chili powder. In a separate medium bowl, whisk the egg.

continued ▶

Chicken Fingers and Cheesy Potatoes *continued*

3. Dredge each chicken tender in the egg and then in the almond flour mixture; then place it on one of the prepared baking sheets. Bake for 10 minutes on the bottom rack; then flip the chicken over and bake for 8 to 10 minutes more, until they're cooked all the way through. If the chicken reaches 165°F internally but is not crispy on the outside, broil for 1 to 5 minutes, watching frequently to prevent burning.

TO MAKE THE POTATOES

4. While the chicken is cooking, cut the potatoes into ¼-inch-thick rounds. In a medium bowl, toss them with the oil, garlic powder, salt, dill, onion powder, and pepper; then spread them out in a single layer on the second prepared baking sheet.

5. Bake for 10 minutes on the top rack; then flip the potatoes over, sprinkle them with Cheddar cheese, and bake for 10 minutes more.

TO SERVE

6. Divide the chicken and potatoes into four servings and serve each with 1 cup of celery sticks and ¼ cup of your favorite sauce for dipping the chicken—try barbecue, ranch, honey mustard, or another delicious dip.

SUBSTITUTION TIP: **Want to add veggies and cut calories and carbs? Use the same amount of seasonings and cheese but slice two large zucchini into rounds instead of the potatoes.**

Per Serving (with low-sugar barbecue sauce)**:** Calories: 431; Fat: 19g; Carbohydrates: 30g; Fiber: 4g; Protein: 39g; Sodium: 1,172mg

Spinach, Red Pepper, and Gruyère Egg Bites

5-ingredient, Gluten-free, Nut-free, Vegetarian
SERVES 4 | **PREP TIME:** 10 minutes | **COOK TIME:** 30 minutes

I love eggs in the morning, but sometimes I get bored with scrambled eggs. Egg bites are the perfect way to get filling protein for breakfast in a convenient package. These egg bites are stuffed with spinach, red pepper, and salty Gruyère cheese for a breakfast you won't want to miss.

Nonstick cooking spray or avocado oil

10 ounces frozen spinach, thawed and squeezed dry (see Substitution Tip)

2 red bell peppers, seeded and diced (see Substitution Tip)

½ cup shredded Gruyère cheese (see Substitution Tip)

8 eggs

1 cup egg whites

¼ teaspoon sea salt (optional)

¼ teaspoon freshly ground black pepper (optional)

1. Preheat the oven to 350°F. Grease a 12-cup muffin tin with nonstick cooking spray or use silicone muffin liners.

2. In a medium bowl, toss together the spinach, bell peppers, and cheese. Fill each muffin cup ½ to ¾ of the way with the mixture.

3. In the same bowl, whisk the eggs, egg whites, and salt and pepper (if using) and divide the mixture among the muffin cups.

4. Bake for 30 minutes, or until the eggs are set. One serving is three egg bites.

SUBSTITUTION TIP: Swap these veggies for chopped zucchini, mushrooms, or any other vegetable you like. You can also change the cheese (Gouda, white Cheddar, Monterey Jack, or Swiss would be delicious) to vary the flavors each time you eat these egg bites.

Per Serving: Calories: 273; Fat: 14g; Carbohydrates: 7g; Fiber: 2g; Protein: 26g; Sodium: 448mg

Soy-Ginger Pork Lettuce Wraps

Dalry-free

SERVES 4 | **PREP TIME:** 10 minutes | **COOK TIME:** 45 minutes

Flavorful stir-fried pork, shredded carrots, and red cabbage are rolled in a lettuce wrap with steamed brown rice. This is my go-to weeknight dinner recipe when I want a healthy meal but don't feel like cooking anything complicated!

3 cups water

1 cup uncooked brown rice (see Cooking Tip)

1 pound lean ground pork (see Substitution Tip)

1 cup shredded carrots

1 cup shredded red cabbage

⅓ cup coconut aminos or soy sauce

1 tablespoon hoisin sauce

1 tablespoon Chinese five-spice powder

½ teaspoon sea salt

½ teaspoon ground ginger

16 butter lettuce leaves

Sriracha (optional)

1. In a medium saucepan over high heat, bring the water to a boil and add the brown rice. Lower the heat to a simmer and cook, covered, for 30 minutes. In a strainer, drain any excess water, add the rice back to the pot, cover, and let stand for 15 minutes. The rice should be chewy and fluffy.

2. While the rice is standing, add the pork to a large nonstick skillet over medium-high heat. Cook for 10 minutes or until the pork is cooked through. Add the shredded carrots, cabbage, coconut aminos, hoisin sauce, five-spice powder, salt, and ginger to the skillet. Stir-fry until the veggies are soft but not mushy, 6 to 8 minutes.

3. Make each wrap using a base of two lettuce leaves on top of each other. Add one-eighth of the brown rice and one-eighth of the pork mixture to each lettuce wrap. Top with some sriracha (if using). One serving is two lettuce wraps.

SUBSTITUTION TIP: **Feel free to use ground turkey or chicken instead of pork.**

COOKING TIP: **To get this recipe time down to less than 30 minutes, use frozen precooked brown rice.**

Per Serving (without the optional Sriracha)**:** Calories: 469; Fat: 20g; Carbohydrates: 46g; Fiber: 3g; Protein: 25g; Sodium: 940mg

Sunshine Lentil Breakfast Bowls

Dairy-free, Gluten-free, Nut-free, Vegetarian
SERVES 4 | **PREP TIME:** 10 minutes | **COOK TIME:** 25 minutes

Sunshine bowls are Buddha bowls that are packed with veggies and topped with soft scrambled or fried eggs for a super filling breakfast. These have the added sunshine of bright orange turmeric tahini sauce. This is the kind of recipe where you can easily vary the veggies you add. You could also use beans instead of lentils or sweet potatoes instead of russet potatoes. The world is your sunshine bowl!

- 2 russet potatoes, cubed
- 3 teaspoons avocado oil, divided
- ½ teaspoon garlic powder
- ½ teaspoon onion powder
- 4 cups chopped asparagus
- 1 teaspoon dried oregano
- 2 tablespoons tahini
- Juice of ½ lemon
- 2 tablespoons maple syrup
- 2 tablespoons water
- ¼ teaspoon ground turmeric
- ¼ teaspoon sea salt
- ¼ teaspoon freshly ground black pepper
- 8 eggs
- 2 cups cooked lentils
- 4 ounces crumbled feta cheese

1. Preheat the oven to 400°F. Line two baking sheets with aluminum foil.

2. Spread the potatoes on one of the prepared baking sheets. Toss with 1½ teaspoons of avocado oil, the garlic powder, and the onion powder. Roast for 20 minutes, until crispy and fork-tender.

3. Meanwhile, add the asparagus to the other baking sheet, toss with the remaining 1½ teaspoons of avocado oil and the oregano, and roast for 15 minutes.

4. While the potatoes and asparagus are roasting, put the tahini, lemon juice, maple syrup, water, turmeric, salt, and pepper in a blender and blend until smooth. Set aside.

5. Scramble or fry two eggs at a time for each serving.

continued ▶

Sunshine Lentil Breakfast Bowls *continued*

6. Assemble each bowl with one-quarter of the cooked lentils, one-quarter of the asparagus, one-quarter of the potatoes, 2 eggs, 1 ounce of crumbled feta cheese, and one-quarter of the sauce. Serve immediately.

> PERFECTLY HEALTHY: **Eggs contain an essential nutrient called choline, which is difficult to obtain elsewhere in the diet, that's linked with improved cognition and brain health. Also, eggs are a great source of protein, which helps keep you fuller for longer to power you through your morning.**

Per Serving: Calories: 559; Fat: 22g; Carbohydrates: 60g; Fiber: 10g; Protein: 34g; Sodium: 534mg

Strawberry Basil Chicken Salad with Baked Goat Cheese

SERVES 4 | **PREP TIME:** 20 minutes | **CHILL TIME:** 35 minutes | **COOK TIME:** 55 minutes

If you've ever been on a diet and eaten a plain chicken salad with vinegar, then you may hate salads. This recipe is here to change the way you think about salads forever. It's packed with flavor from sweet, succulent strawberries, fresh basil, tangy walnut-crusted baked goat cheese, juicy chicken, and a fresh, easy balsamic honey dressing. If you aren't assembling the salad to eat right away, store the chicken, basil, goat cheese balls, and dressing separately to assemble later.

Nonstick cooking spray or avocado oil

½ cup shelled walnuts

½ cup panko bread crumbs

1 teaspoon sea salt, divided

1 (8-ounce) log honey goat cheese

1 egg, whisked

1½ pounds boneless, skinless chicken breast, diced

¼ teaspoon freshly ground black pepper

¼ cup extra-virgin olive oil

¼ cup balsamic vinegar

2 tablespoons honey

¼ cup water

8 cups mixed greens

4 cups strawberries, quartered

½ cup chopped fresh basil

1. Line a baking sheet with parchment paper and spray with nonstick cooking spray or grease with avocado oil.

2. In a food processor, process the walnuts until they're coarse but not as fine as flour. In a medium bowl, mix the ground nuts with the bread crumbs and ½ teaspoon of salt.

3. Cut the goat cheese into 12 slices and roll them into balls. Dip the goat cheese balls into the whisked egg and then into the bread crumb mixture. Place the balls on the lined baking sheet. Freeze for 35 minutes.

4. While the goat cheese is chilling, preheat the oven to 375°F. Line a baking sheet with aluminum foil and spray with nonstick cooking spray or grease with avocado oil.

continued ▶

Strawberry Basil Chicken Salad with Baked Goat Cheese *continued*

5. Spread the chicken on the second baking sheet and toss with the remaining ½ teaspoon of salt and the pepper. Bake for 35 to 45 minutes, until no pink remains and the internal temperature reaches 165°F.

6. Raise the oven temperature to 450°F. Bake the cheese balls (straight out of the freezer) for 6 to 8 minutes, until they are golden brown and crispy.

7. While the cheese balls are baking, in a small bowl, combine the olive oil, vinegar, honey, and water and whisk well until thoroughly mixed.

8. Assemble each salad with 2 cups of mixed greens, 1 cup of fresh strawberries, one-quarter of the chicken, and 3 tablespoons of the dressing. Add 3 goat cheese balls to each salad and top with 2 tablespoons of fresh basil. Serve.

> LEFTOVER TIP: **You will have about ⅔ cup of the walnut and bread crumb mixture and half the egg mixture leftover; this is not included in the nutrition information. You won't be able to save this because it will be contaminated with raw egg. However, you could get more goat cheese and freeze extra balls to cook the next time you make this recipe.**

Per Serving: Calories: 668; Fat: 34g; Carbohydrates: 38g; Fiber: 4g; Protein: 51g; Sodium: 450mg

Broiled Sweet and Peppery Steak with Asparagus

Dairy-free, Gluten-free, Nut-free, Sheet pan
SERVES 4 | **PREP TIME:** 10 minutes | **COOK TIME:** 30 minutes

Broiling steak is one of my favorite ways to cook it because it's just so easy. This steak is broiled to perfection with a sweet and peppery rub and then served with roasted asparagus for a delicious and simple meal that comes together in no time.

Nonstick cooking spray or avocado oil

1 tablespoon coconut sugar

1 teaspoon sea salt

1 teaspoon freshly ground black pepper

½ teaspoon onion flakes

½ teaspoon garlic powder

½ teaspoon smoked paprika

¼ teaspoon red pepper flakes

4 (8-ounce) 100 percent grass-fed flatiron steaks (see Perfectly Healthy note)

1½ pounds asparagus

2 teaspoons avocado oil

1 teaspoon garlic salt

½ teaspoon lemon pepper

1. Preheat the broiler. Line two baking sheets with aluminum foil and spray with nonstick cooking spray.

2. In a small bowl, combine the coconut sugar, salt, pepper, onion flakes, garlic powder, paprika, and red pepper flakes. Rub the mixture all over the steaks, covering as much of them as possible.

3. Put the steaks on one of the prepared baking sheets and broil to your desired doneness, flipping the steaks over about halfway through the cooking time. For medium, it will take 12 to 15 minutes. Broil times may vary depending on the thickness of the steak and how you like them cooked. Transfer the steaks to a cutting board and let them rest for 15 minutes before slicing.

4. Turn the oven to 400°F.

5. Add the asparagus to the other baking sheet and toss with the oil, garlic salt, and lemon pepper. Roast for 15 minutes; the asparagus is done when it is fork-tender. Serve immediately.

continued ▶

Broiled Sweet and Peppery Steak with Asparagus *continued*

PERFECTLY HEALTHY: **One hundred percent grass-fed meat is high in anti-oxidants and anti-inflammatory omega-3 fats, so if your budget permits, it's the healthiest type of meat to buy. If you can't find it or it doesn't fit in your budget, get the leanest cut of meat possible and cut any visible fat from the meat.**

Per Serving: Calories: 437; Fat: 21g; Carbohydrates: 8g; Fiber: 2g; Protein: 51g; Sodium: 1,383mg

Spanakopita Veggie Burgers with Mixed Greens

Nut-free, Sheet pan, Vegetarian
SERVES 4 | **PREP TIME:** 10 minutes | **COOK TIME:** 25 minutes

These veggie burgers are inspired by the classic Greek dish spanakopita, which packs spinach and feta into a buttery pastry layer. While there is no pastry here, the burgers do bake in the oven to a crispy golden-brown perfection and are packed with spinach and salty feta cheese in every bite.

2 cups cooked lentils

¾ cup crumbled feta cheese

10 ounces frozen spinach, thawed and squeezed dry

2 eggs

½ cup whole-wheat bread crumbs

¼ teaspoon sea salt

4 cups mixed greens

¼ cup salad dressing (of your choice)

1. Preheat the oven to 350°F. Line a baking sheet with parchment paper.

2. In a food processor, combine the lentils, feta, spinach, eggs, bread crumbs, and salt. Pulse to mix. Form the mixture into eight patties using about ¼ cup of the mixture per patty.

3. Put the patties on the prepared baking sheet and bake for 20 to 25 minutes, until warmed through and firm.

4. Each serving is two patties, 1 cup of mixed greens, and 1 tablespoon of your favorite salad dressing.

LEFTOVER TIP: Store the burgers in the refrigerator for up to 5 days or freeze them for up to 3 months. If you freeze them, you can reheat them from frozen in the microwave or thaw them in the refrigerator and quickly pan-fry to crisp them up.

Per Serving (without salad dressing)**:** Calories: 337; Fat: 10g; Carbohydrates: 40g; Fiber: 7g; Protein: 23g; Sodium: 676mg

Orange Dreamsicle Protein Smoothie

Gluten-free, No-cook, Nut-free, Vegetarian
SERVES 2 | **PREP TIME:** 10 minutes | **CHILL TIME:** overnight

My husband lives for those orange cream ice pops of our childhood—the ones with the bright orange outside and creamy sweet center. This smoothie tastes like those orange delights but is healthy enough for breakfast. I make this whenever I want a slam-dunk breakfast in smoothie form for the hubby, and I know you'll love it too.

2 navel oranges, peeled and cut into wedges

1 banana, peeled and cut into chunks (see Substitution Tip)

½ cup vanilla protein powder

1½ cups unsweetened almond milk

¼ teaspoon orange extract (see Cooking Tip)

1 teaspoon vanilla extract

1. Slice and freeze the oranges and banana the night before. Freeze the orange wedges on a wax or parchment paper–lined pan or dish so they don't stick together in one frozen clump.

2. The next morning, in a blender, blend the oranges, banana, protein powder, milk, orange extract, and vanilla extract until smooth. Serve immediately.

SUBSTITUTION TIP: **If you don't love bananas, substitute two pitted dates for natural sweetness and ½ cup of ice.**

COOKING TIP: **Look for orange extract near the vanilla extract in the supermarket.**

Per Serving: Calories: 230; Fat: 3g; Carbohydrates: 33g; Fiber: 6g; Protein: 22g; Sodium: 160mg

Green Chile Beef Tacos with Cherry Tomato Salad

30 minutes or less

SERVES 4 | **PREP TIME:** 10 minutes | **COOK TIME:** 20 minutes

I love taco night, and so does my family. I feel like anytime I propose "build your own" anything, everybody gets excited. This isn't your average taco meat either. It's packed with diced tomatoes and roasted green chiles for a flavorful filling that is guaranteed to not leave you hungry. Serve it with a crunchy tomato salad and homemade salsa for a delicious fiesta dinner.

½ **tablespoon avocado oil**

½ **yellow onion, chopped**

2 **garlic cloves, minced**

1 **pound 90 percent lean ground beef** (see Substitution Tip)

¼ **cup taco seasoning**

1 **(15-ounce) can diced tomatoes, drained**

1 **(4-ounce) can green chiles, drained**

4 **cups cherry tomatoes, halved**

1 **tablespoon extra-virgin olive oil**

1 **tablespoon balsamic vinegar**

½ **teaspoon garlic salt**

½ **teaspoon freshly ground black pepper**

8 **(6-inch) corn tortillas**

½ **cup shredded Cheddar cheese**

1 **cup shredded green cabbage**

Fresh Homemade Salsa, for garnish (optional; page 62)

1. In a large nonstick skillet over medium-high heat, heat the avocado oil, add the onion and garlic, and cook for 1 to 2 minutes, until they're translucent and tender. Add the ground beef and taco seasoning and cook for 10 minutes, breaking up the beef with a wooden spoon, until cooked through. Add the diced tomatoes and green chiles and let simmer for 3 to 5 minutes, until most of the liquid has evaporated.

2. In a medium bowl, gently toss the cherry tomatoes with the olive oil, vinegar, garlic salt, and pepper.

continued ▶

Green Chile Beef Tacos with Cherry Tomato Salad *continued*

3. Divide the meat mixture into eight servings. Assemble eight tacos by spooning one portion of the meat mixture onto each tortilla, followed by 1 tablespoon of cheese and 2 tablespoons of green cabbage plus some salsa (if using). A serving is two tacos and one-quarter of the tomato salad.

SUBSTITUTION TIP: **Use ground turkey or ground chicken to change the flavor or to lighten up this meal a bit.**

COOKING TIP: **If you are serving this as a family meal, serve it with all the traditional taco bar fixings to provide variety for everyone.**

Per Serving (without Fresh Homemade Salsa)**:** Calories: 547; Fat: 24g; Carbohydrates: 46g; Fiber: 5g; Protein: 35g; Sodium: 508mg

Black Bean Breakfast Burritos

30 minutes or less, Nut-free, Vegetarian
SERVES 4 | **PREP TIME:** 10 minutes | **COOK TIME:** 15 minutes

It took me a long time to realize that breakfast burritos didn't just mean going to the drive-through the morning after a long night in college (studying, of course). Hangover or not, I can make a healthy breakfast burrito at home anytime I want. These burritos have enough protein and fiber to power you through your morning.

½ **tablespoon avocado oil**

½ **yellow onion, chopped**

2 **garlic cloves, minced**

1 **(15-ounce) can diced tomatoes, drained**

1 **(15-ounce) can black beans, drained and rinsed**

8 **eggs**

¼ **teaspoon sea salt**

¼ **teaspoon freshly ground black pepper**

1 **tablespoon salted butter**

4 **(10-inch) whole-wheat tortillas**

½ **cup shredded Monterey Jack cheese**

Fresh Homemade Salsa, for garnish (optional; page 62)

1. In a large nonstick skillet over medium-high heat, heat the oil and cook the onion and garlic for 1 to 2 minutes, until they're translucent and tender. Add the diced tomatoes and black beans and simmer for 3 to 5 minutes, until most of the liquid has evaporated.

2. In a medium bowl, whisk the eggs with the salt and pepper.

3. In a medium nonstick skillet over medium heat, heat the butter. When the butter is melted and bubbly, add the eggs and scramble until they are fully set.

4. To each tortilla, add one-quarter of the black bean mixture, one-quarter of the eggs, and 2 tablespoons of cheese. Roll up the burritos and serve with some salsa on the side (if using).

LEFTOVER TIP: Store the leftover egg mixture separately from the remaining tortillas so that the tortillas don't get soggy. Roll the burritos right before you are ready to eat them.

Per Serving (without Fresh Homemade Salsa)**:** Calories: 544; Fat: 27g; Carbohydrates: 46g; Fiber: 12g; Protein: 31g; Sodium: 839mg

Vegan Thai-Style Curry

**30 minutes or less, 5-ingredient, Dairy-free,
Gluten-free, Nut-free, One pot, Vegan**
SERVES 4 | **PREP TIME:** 5 minutes | **COOK TIME:** 20 minutes

This vegan Thai-style curry brings frozen veggies to life with a little spice and a whole lot of creaminess. The best part is you need only five ingredients to get dinner on the table. I mean, there pretty much isn't anything better than that!

**2 tablespoons
sesame oil**

**1 pound high-protein
or extra-firm tofu,
cut into cubes** (see
Substitution Tip)

**6 cups frozen stir-fry
vegetable mix**

2 cups Thai curry sauce

**2 cups cooked
brown rice**

1. In a large nonstick skillet over medium-high heat, heat the oil and stir-fry the tofu until crispy and golden brown all over, 8 to 12 minutes. Remove the tofu from the skillet and set aside.

2. Put the frozen veggies in the same pan, cover the pan, and cook, stirring occasionally, until fully defrosted, 5 to 7 minutes. Drain any excess liquid.

3. Add the curry sauce to the veggies, cover the pan, and let the mixture simmer for 10 minutes, until the veggies are fork-tender. Add the tofu back to the pan.

4. Divide the curry into four portions and serve each portion over ½ cup of brown rice.

SUBSTITUTION TIP: **Feel free to change the protein in this recipe to give it a different taste. I love to use cooked cubed chicken or shrimp.**

Per Serving: Calories: 565; Fat: 28g; Carbohydrates: 51g; Fiber: 9g; Protein: 24g; Sodium: 569mg

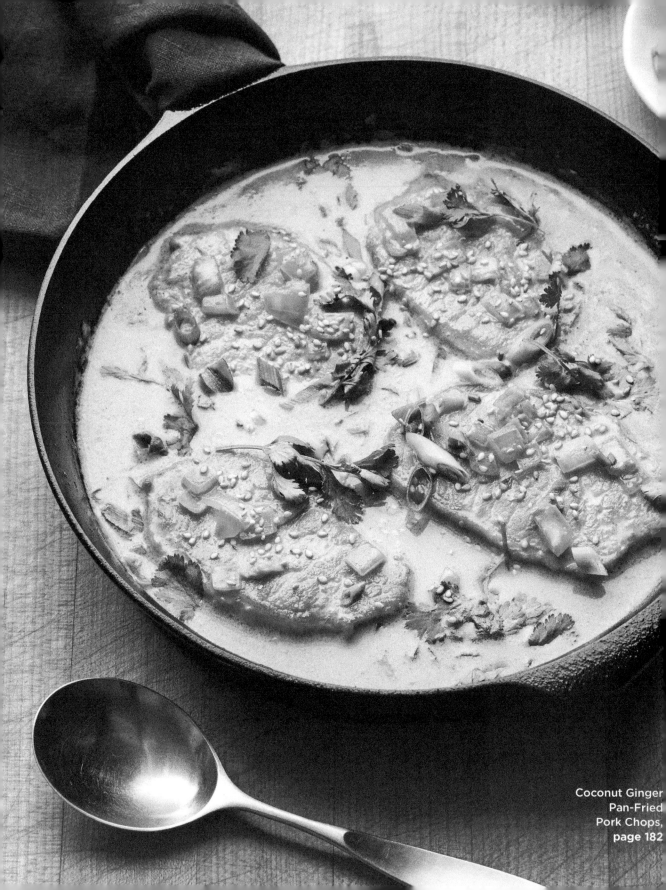

Coconut Ginger
Pan-Fried
Pork Chops,
page 182

CHAPTER 8

Bonus Healthy Recipes for Life

YOUR HEALTHY WEIGHT LOSS JOURNEY DOESN'T HAVE to end with the 30-day plan. Use the following recipes to create your own weekly plans using the information you've learned over the past 30 days.

Breakfasts

Easy Spinach Scrambled Eggs on Avocado Toast

30 minutes or less, 5-ingredient, Dairy-free, Nut-free, Vegetarian
SERVES 4 | **PREP TIME:** 5 minutes | **COOK TIME:** 10 minutes

Nothing beats the simplicity and deliciousness of creamy scrambled eggs on toast. Add in mashed avocado with a sprinkle of everything bagel seasoning, and you're guaranteed to be in breakfast heaven. Remember, avocados are not bad for you! In fact, they are probably one of the healthiest foods you could eat. They are packed with vitamins, minerals, fiber, and heart-healthy fats that keep you full. I recommend that my clients eat at least half an avocado a day.

2 large slices whole-grain bread

½ avocado, mashed, divided

4 eggs

Nonstick cooking spray

2 cups spinach

1 teaspoon everything bagel seasoning, divided

1. Toast the bread slices. When the toast is ready, spread half the mashed avocado on each piece.

2. In a small bowl, whisk the eggs.

3. Spray a medium nonstick skillet with nonstick cooking spray. Put in the spinach and sauté over medium heat until just wilted, about 2 minutes. Pour the eggs over the wilted spinach. Scramble the eggs until they're cooked the way you like.

4. Add half the egg mixture to each piece of toast. Sprinkle each piece with ½ teaspoon of everything bagel seasoning and serve.

> COOKING TIP: **Scrambled eggs can vary from a soft scramble to fully cooked. For a soft scramble, gently fold in the edges until the eggs are just set but still glistening. For fully cooked eggs, continue to cook them until they are no longer glistening and are completely dry.**

Per Serving: Calories: 385; Fat: 22g; Carbohydrates: 31g; Fiber: 6g; Protein: 18g; Sodium: 524mg

Soft Scrambled Eggs and Roasted Veggies

Dairy-free, Gluten-free, Nut-free, Vegetarian
SERVES 4 | **PREP TIME:** 10 minutes | **COOK TIME:** 25 minutes

Soft-scrambling eggs is a technique that creates soft, luxurious eggs that taste rich and creamy. To soft-scramble your eggs, pour them in the skillet and then slowly push the spatula from the outside in, creating soft ribbons around the skillet. They are done when they're firm but still shiny. The creamy texture of these eggs pairs perfectly with the roasted broccoli and potatoes for a colorful and delicious breakfast. Serve with Fresh Home-made Salsa (page 62), ketchup, or whatever you like with your eggs.

2 large purple sweet potatoes, cut into 1-inch cubes

½ teaspoon cinnamon

1 tablespoon maple syrup

1 tablespoon coconut oil, melted

Nonstick cooking spray

2 cups broccoli florets

¼ teaspoon sea salt

¼ teaspoon freshly ground black pepper

8 eggs, divided

1 cup egg whites, divided

1. Preheat the oven to 400°F. Line two baking sheets with aluminum foil. Set one rack in the bottom of your oven and one in the top.

2. In a large bowl, toss the sweet potatoes with the cinnamon, maple syrup, and coconut oil. Spread them on one of the prepared baking sheets. Place it on the bottom rack and bake for 20 minutes.

3. Spray the second sheet with nonstick cooking spray, spread out the broccoli on the sheet, and spray the florets with more cooking oil. Sprinkle with the salt and pepper, and then bake for 15 minutes or until fork-tender.

4. In a small bowl, whisk 2 eggs and ¼ cup of egg whites.

5. Spray a medium nonstick skillet with nonstick cooking spray. Set it over medium heat and soft-scramble the eggs.

6. Spoon one-quarter of the sweet potatoes, one-quarter of the broccoli, and one-quarter of the eggs onto each of four plates.

PERFECTLY HEALTHY: **Purple sweet potatoes are a fun variation on the typical orange sweet potato. The purple color comes from the abundant anthocyanins, an antioxidant shown to help reduce blood pressure, inflammation levels, and the risk of diabetes and cancer.**

Per Serving: Calories: 292; Fat: 13g; Carbohydrates: 21g; Fiber: 3g; Protein: 22g; Sodium: 441mg

Super Seed Loaded Oats

30 minutes or less, Gluten-free, Nut-free, Vegetarian
SERVES 4 | **PREP TIME:** 5 minutes | **COOK TIME:** 10 minutes

This recipe uses steel-cut oats—oats that have been chopped into pieces instead of rolled out flat, as we are used to seeing with rolled oats. All oats are good for you, but because of the way they are processed, steel-cut oats have slightly more fiber and nutrients than rolled oats. The seeds in this oatmeal really complement the chewy, hearty texture of steel-cut oats.

2¼ cups water

¾ cup quick-cooking steel-cut oats

½ cup hemp seeds

⅓ cup ground flaxseed

⅓ cup pumpkin seeds

1 teaspoon cinnamon

¾ cup unsweetened almond milk or other unsweetened milk

4 tablespoons raisins, divided

2 tablespoons honey, divided

2 ripe bananas, sliced, divided

1. In a medium saucepan over high heat, bring the water to a boil, and then add the oats. Reduce the heat to medium and cook for 7 to 9 minutes, until most of the liquid is absorbed and the oats are tender.

2. Stir in the hemp seeds, flaxseed, pumpkin seeds, and cinnamon. Add the milk as needed to reach the desired creaminess, up to ¾ cup.

3. Divide the oatmeal into four bowls and top with 1 tablespoon of raisins, 1½ teaspoons of honey, and half a sliced banana.

PERFECTLY HEALTHY: Super seeds like hemp seed hearts, ground flax, and others have gained a reputation for being nutritional powerhouses because they are rich in protein, heart-healthy fats, and inflammation-fighting antioxidants.

Per Serving: Calories: 482; Fat: 22g; Carbohydrates: 62g; Fiber: 9g; Protein: 16g; Sodium: 26mg

Southwest Egg Bites

Gluten-free, Nut-free, Vegetarian
SERVES 4 | **PREP TIME:** 15 minutes | **COOK TIME:** 40 minutes

The inspiration for these egg bites was the leftover jalapeño peppers, cream cheese, and sour cream I had in the refrigerator after making bacon jalapeño poppers one weekend. I decided to turn the leftover ingredients into delicious, healthy egg bites that are full of flavor. If you have sensitive skin, I recommend wearing gloves to protect your hands and avoid touching your face or anything else while handling jalapeños.

Nonstick cooking spray

1 teaspoon avocado oil

1 jalapeño pepper, deveined, seeded, and chopped

1 zucchini, diced

½ yellow onion, chopped

1 garlic clove, minced

6 eggs

¾ cup egg whites

¼ cup sour cream

½ cup whipped cream cheese

½ cup shredded Cheddar cheese

½ teaspoon chili powder

1. Preheat the oven to 375°F. Grease a 12-cup muffin tin with nonstick cooking spray.

2. In a medium nonstick skillet over medium-high heat, heat the avocado oil. Add the jalapeño, zucchini, onion, and garlic and cook for 5 to 7 minutes, until translucent and tender. Divide the veggies evenly among the muffin cups.

3. Combine the eggs, egg whites, sour cream, cream cheese, Cheddar cheese, and chili powder in a blender and blend until well mixed. Divide the mixture among the muffin cups, pouring the egg mixture on top of the veggies.

4. Bake for 30 minutes, until the eggs are set. Serve.

PERFECTLY HEALTHY: Jalapeño peppers are rich in vitamins A and C and potassium. Most of their health benefits come from capsaicin, which is actively being researched for its potential to fight cancer and ward off chronic diseases. It also gives the body a very slight metabolism boost, which, although it is short-lived, is never a bad thing.

Per Serving: Calories: 262; Fat: 20g; Carbohydrates: 5g; Fiber: 1g; Protein: 15g; Sodium: 309mg

Hemp Seed Muffins

Nut-free, Vegetarian
SERVES 12 | **PREP TIME:** 5 minutes | **COOK TIME:** 30 minutes

Hemp seeds are packed with protein, healthy fat, and fiber, making these muffins more filling than your standard breakfast muffin. Whole-wheat flour replaces refined white flour, and coconut sugar stands in for processed refined sugar for a nutrient boost. And for a nice surprise, these muffins have a sweet crust on top and are moist on the inside, with just a hint of nuttiness from the hemp seeds.

Nonstick cooking spray or avocado oil

1½ cups whole-wheat pastry flour

1 cup hemp seeds

¾ cup coconut sugar

¾ cup unsweetened almond milk or other unsweetened milk

½ cup unsweetened applesauce

2 eggs

1 teaspoon cinnamon

1 teaspoon baking powder

½ teaspoon baking soda

⅛ teaspoon sea salt

1. Preheat the oven to 350°F. Grease a 12-cup muffin tin with nonstick cooking spray.

2. Combine the flour, hemp seeds, coconut sugar, milk, applesauce, eggs, cinnamon, baking powder, baking soda, and salt in a food processor or blender and blend until smooth.

3. Divide the ingredients evenly among the muffin tin cups and bake for 30 minutes, or until a toothpick inserted in the center of one muffin comes out clean. Serve.

LEFTOVER TIP: **Store these muffins in the refrigerator for up to 1 week or freeze them for up to 3 months.**

Per Serving: Calories: 172; Fat: 8g; Carbohydrates: 23g; Fiber: 3g; Protein: 7g; Sodium: 132mg

Cinnamon Spice Almond Flour Pancakes

30 minutes or less, Dairy-free, Gluten-free, Vegetarian
SERVES 3 | **PREP TIME:** 5 minutes | **COOK TIME:** 15 minutes

Pancake lovers, this one is for you! I love using almond flour in baked goods because it is packed with protein, healthy fat, and fiber that wheat flour doesn't provide. These pancakes are more filling and also more flavorful than most pancakes. The idea for these came to me when my hubby was going through a chai tea latte obsession, so I filled pancakes with chai tea spices, and he was even more obsessed! I know you'll enjoy these fluffy pancakes too.

1⅓ cup almond flour

¼ cup unsweetened vanilla almond milk

3 eggs

1 teaspoon baking powder

2 tablespoons coconut sugar

2 teaspoon cinnamon (see Cooking Tip)

½ teaspoon ground nutmeg (see Cooking Tip)

½ teaspoon ground allspice (see Cooking Tip)

⅛ teaspoon sea salt

Nonstick cooking spray or avocado oil

Almond Butter Syrup (optional; page 80)

1. Combine the almond flour, almond milk, eggs, baking powder, coconut sugar, cinnamon, nutmeg, allspice, and salt in a blender and blend just until smooth. Make sure you don't overmix the batter.

2. Heat a nonstick skillet over medium heat and spray with nonstick cooking spray. Cook ¼ cup of batter at a time. Cook each pancake for 2 to 3 minutes, until you see bubbles on the top; then flip it over and cook for 2 to 3 minutes more.

3. A serving is two pancakes. Top them with Almond Butter Syrup, if you'd like.

continued ▶

Cinnamon Spice Almond Flour Pancakes *continued*

COOKING TIP: If you don't love spicy chai flavor, halve the amount of spices for a milder flavor to your pancake.

LEFTOVER TIP: Pancakes stay fresh for 3 days in the refrigerator, or you can freeze them for up to 3 months. If you freeze them, place a piece of wax paper or parchment paper in between each to keep them from sticking, and then you can defrost just one or two at a time.

Per Serving (without the optional Almond Butter Syrup)**:** Calories: 377; Fat: 30g; Carbohydrates: 17g; Fiber: 5g; Protein: 17g; Sodium: 296mg

Bacon and Eggs Healthy Breakfast Sandwiches

30 minutes or less, Nut-free
SERVES 4 | **PREP TIME:** 10 minutes | **COOK TIME:** 20 minutes

Bacon? In a healthy weight loss cookbook? Although I didn't use it in the other recipes, mostly because it's a hassle to cook and increases the cooking time of a recipe, I wanted to put it in at least once. Sure, bacon isn't the healthiest food in the world because it's high in sodium and saturated fat, but in thoughtful portions, it can fit in a balanced diet. This egg and bacon breakfast sandwich is also packed with nutrient-dense foods such as avocado, tomato, and sprouts.

4 slices bacon (see Perfectly Healthy note)

4 whole-grain English muffins

Nonstick cooking spray

8 eggs

¼ cup whipped cream cheese, divided

1 avocado, sliced, divided

1 tomato, sliced, divided

1 cup bean sprouts, divided

1 teaspoon everything bagel seasoning, divided

1. In a medium skillet over medium heat, cook the bacon for 8 to 10 minutes, until crispy all over. Drain and blot the bacon on paper towels.

2. While the bacon is cooking, toast the English muffins until they're golden brown.

3. Spray a large skillet with nonstick cooking spray and fry or scramble the eggs over medium heat until they are done the way you like them.

4. Spread 1 tablespoon of cream cheese on one side of each muffin; then add one-quarter of the avocado slices, 1 piece of bacon, one-quarter of the tomato slices, ¼ cup of sprouts, 2 eggs (if fried) or one-quarter of the eggs (if scrambled), and ¼ teaspoon of everything bagel seasoning. Top with the other side of the English muffin and dig in!

Bacon and Eggs Healthy Breakfast Sandwiches *continued*

> PERFECTLY HEALTHY: When shopping for bacon or any type of processed meat, such as deli meat, choose nitrate-free or uncured versions. Conventional bacon includes nitrates and nitrites as preservatives, which have been strongly linked to an increased risk of cancer. It's unclear whether processed meat that is uncured raises any health risk, since it hasn't been widely studied, so it's best to get uncured nitrate-free versions to avoid preservatives and chemicals as much as possible.

Per Serving: Calories: 436; Fat: 25g; Carbohydrates: 30g; Fiber: 7g; Protein: 7g; Sodium: 691mg

Peanut Butter Banana Green Smoothie

30 minutes or less, Dairy-free, Gluten-free, No-cook, Vegan
SERVES 2 | **PREP TIME:** 10 minutes

Peanut butter and banana is my favorite flavor combination in a smoothie. I used both peanut butter powder and peanut butter to make this extra peanut buttery and to add more protein without packing in excess calories. It's the perfect nutritional and flavor balance for a delicious morning smoothie, and you won't even taste the greens.

2 frozen bananas

1 cup ice

1 cup unsweetened vanilla almond milk

⅓ cup peanut butter powder

2 tablespoons peanut butter

4 cups spinach

Vanilla liquid stevia drops

Place the bananas, almond milk, peanut butter powder, peanut butter, spinach, and stevia in a blender and blend until smooth. Serve immediately.

> **PERFECTLY HEALTHY:** Peanut butter powder is not necessarily better or worse than peanut butter. It's all about what type of meal you are trying to create. Remember, each meal should have protein, fat, veggies, and varying amounts of complex carbs. The peanut butter by itself does not raise the protein content high enough to keep you full and promote weight loss, but it does provide some healthy fat. So by using a combination of fat-free peanut butter powder and real peanut butter, you get the best of both worlds and an ultra–peanut butter breakfast shake!

Per Serving: Calories: 309; Fat: 12g; Carbohydrates: 40g; Fiber: 7g; Protein: 15g; Sodium: 252mg

Vegetarian and Seafood Entrées

Lentil Tahini Burgers

Dairy-free, Nut-free, Vegetarian
SERVES 4 | **PREP TIME:** 15 minutes | **CHILL TIME:** 1 hour | **COOK TIME:** 10 minutes

If you are new to incorporating vegetarian recipes into your weekly rotation, don't think of these as a burger replacement. Nothing replaces a burger. Instead, think of them as a fun and delicious way to include more healthy foods in your diet. We eat these with lettuce wraps and lots of fixings, such as ketchup, mustard, onions, tomatoes, and relish.

½ **large red onion, diced**

2 **garlic cloves, diced**

3 **tablespoons avocado oil, divided**

2 **cups cooked black lentils, divided**

½ **cup tahini**

½ **cup whole-wheat bread crumbs**

¼ **cup rolled oats**

2 **eggs**

½ **teaspoon dried oregano**

½ **teaspoon dried basil**

¼ **teaspoon ground cumin**

1 **teaspoon smoked paprika**

Freshly ground black pepper

1. In a food processor, pulse the red onion and garlic until they're finely diced.

2. In a medium skillet over medium-high heat, heat 1 teaspoon of oil; then add the onion and garlic. Cook for 1 to 2 minutes, until the onion is translucent and tender and the garlic is fragrant.

3. In the food processor, combine 1 cup of lentils, the tahini, bread crumbs, oats, eggs, oregano, basil, cumin, paprika, pepper, and the onion and garlic mixture. Process until everything is combined but not liquid. Stir the remaining 1 cup of lentils into the mixture.

4. Form the mixture into palm-size patties and place them on a plate. Refrigerate for 1 hour.

5. In a large skillet, heat the remaining 2 tablespoons of oil. Pan-fry the patties on medium heat for 3 to 5 minutes on each side, until they're golden brown on both sides and heated through. Serve.

| PERFECTLY HEALTHY: **Lentils offer high protein, fiber, and nutrient content.**

Per Serving: Calories: 540; Fat: 31g; Carbohydrates: 47g; Fiber: 8g; Protein: 23g; Sodium: 175mg

Sweet and Sour Chickpea Bowls

30 minutes or less, Dairy-free, Gluten-free, Nut-free, Vegan
SERVES 4 | **PREP TIME:** 5 minutes | **COOK TIME:** 20 minutes

This is a fun vegetarian spin on a classic Chinese takeout dish. The sweet and sour sauce is a little higher in carbohydrates, as are the chickpeas, so I would skip rice or use cauliflower rice to keep the carb count in check. We typically don't serve this with anything and eat it as is because it's so delicious and filling. It's sweet yet sour and packed with flavor in every bite.

1 tablespoon avocado oil

6 cups frozen stir-fry vegetables (see Substitution Tip)

⅓ cup coconut sugar

¼ cup apple cider vinegar

2 tablespoons ketchup

2 tablespoons orange juice

2 tablespoons coconut aminos or soy sauce

1 tablespoon tomato paste

1½ teaspoons water

1 teaspoon cornstarch

2 tablespoons sesame oil

2 (15-ounce) cans chickpeas, drained and rinsed

1. In a large skillet over medium-high heat, heat the oil. Add the frozen stir fry veggies and cook for 7 to 10 minutes, until they're hot throughout and softened.

2. Meanwhile, in a small saucepan over medium heat, combine the coconut sugar, vinegar, ketchup, orange juice, coconut aminos, tomato paste, water, and cornstarch. Whisk well to combine and bring to a slow boil. Let simmer for 10 minutes until thickened.

3. When the veggies are warm, remove them from the skillet and put in the sesame oil and chickpeas. Sauté the chickpeas until they're slightly browned and crunchy.

4. Add the heated veggies and the sauce to the skillet with the chickpeas and combine. Serve.

SUBSTITUTION TIP: **You can use your own combo of fresh vegetables instead of frozen or 6 cups of mixed broccoli, carrots, bell peppers, and snow peas.**

Per Serving: Calories: 307; Fat: 7g; Carbohydrates: 49g; Fiber: 11g; Protein: 11g; Sodium: 176mg

Bean and Cheese Taquitos

5-ingredient, Nut-free, Sheet pan, Vegetarian
SERVES 4 | **PREP TIME:** 10 minutes | **COOK TIME:** 25 minutes

These taquitos are baked instead of deep-fried, saving thousands of calories. My family *loves* these crunchy, cheesy stuffed taquitos, and I love serving them because they use just five ingredients. For a veggie to go with this meal, I love a bowl of taco-seasoned cauliflower rice or a simple side salad.

Nonstick cooking spray

12 (6-inch) corn tortillas

½ (15-ounce) can refried beans, divided

1 (4-ounce) can green chiles, drained, divided

1½ cups shredded Monterey Jack cheese, divided (see Substitution Tip)

1 (10-ounce) block frozen spinach, thawed and squeezed dry, divided

¼ teaspoon sea salt

1. Preheat the oven to 425°F. Line one baking sheet with aluminum foil and spray it with nonstick cooking spray. Line another baking sheet with parchment paper and spray it with nonstick cooking spray.

2. Spread the tortillas on the foil-lined baking sheet in two overlapping rows. Bake them until they're hot, about 2 minutes. Transfer the tortillas to a plate and cover them with a clean kitchen towel.

3. Place six tortillas on a clean work surface. Working quickly, spread ½ tablespoon of refried beans, ½ tablespoon of green chiles, 2 tablespoons of cheese, and 2 tablespoons of spinach on each tortilla. Roll into a tight cigar shape. Transfer to the parchment-lined baking sheet. Repeat with the remaining six tortillas.

4. Generously coat the tops and sides of the taquitos with nonstick cooking spray. Sprinkle the tops with the salt. Bake the taquitos until they're browned and crispy, 18 to 24 minutes. One serving is three taquitos.

SUBSTITUTION TIP: **You can also use other types of cheese, such as shredded Mexican cheese blend, for a slightly different flavor.**

COOKING TIP: **This recipe will work in the air fryer as well. Preheat your air fryer to 400°F and cook for 6 to 12 minutes, flipping the taquitos halfway through.**

Per Serving: Calories: 622; Fat: 30g; Carbohydrates: 55g; Fiber: 8g; Protein: 29g; Sodium: 775mg

Green Goddess Tofu Bowls

Dairy-free, Gluten-free, Nut-free, Vegetarian
SERVES 4 | **PREP TIME:** 10 minutes | **COOK TIME:** 45 minutes

This might be one of my favorite recipes of all time. It's filling and warm, packed with roasted veggies and baked tofu and then drizzled with this delightful lemony sauce, all served over a bed of wild rice. You can easily make this vegan by choosing a vegan mayonnaise for the dressing.

FOR THE BOWLS

Nonstick cooking spray or avocado oil

1 cup wild rice

1¾ cups water

1 pound high-protein tofu, sliced into 1-inch-thick slices

Sea salt

Freshly ground black pepper

2 cup Brussels sprouts, halved

2 cups broccoli florets

4 cups fresh spinach

FOR THE GREEN GODDESS DRESSING

½ cup fresh parsley, stems removed

½ cup spinach

1 scallion, roughly chopped

1 garlic clove

1 tablespoon soy sauce or coconut aminos

¼ cup freshly squeezed lemon juice

2 tablespoon extra-virgin olive oil

½ teaspoon sea salt

¼ cup avocado oil mayonnaise

TO MAKE THE BOWLS

1. Preheat the oven to 400°F. Line two baking sheets with aluminum foil and spray both with nonstick cooking spray.

2. Put the wild rice and water in a small pot and bring to a boil over high heat. Reduce the heat to medium, cover, and simmer for 40 to 45 minutes, until all the water is absorbed.

3. While the rice is cooking, spread out the tofu on one of the prepared baking sheets. Sprinkle ¼ teaspoon of salt and some pepper on the top of each piece; then spray it with nonstick cooking spray. Bake for 20 minutes, flipping the pieces halfway through.

4. Meanwhile, on the second prepared baking sheet, spread out the Brussels sprouts and broccoli and spray with nonstick cooking spray. Bake for 15 to 20 minutes, until fork-tender.

5. Assemble each bowl with ½ cup of cooked rice, 1 cup of spinach, one-quarter of the tofu slices, and 1 cup each of the Brussels sprouts and broccoli.

TO MAKE THE DRESSING

6. While everything is in the oven, make the dressing by combining the parsley, spinach, scallion, garlic, soy sauce, lemon juice, olive oil, and salt in a high-powered blender or food processor. Blend until well combined.

7. To the blender, add the mayo and blend again for 5 to 10 seconds.

8. Drizzle each bowl with one-quarter of the green goddess dressing and serve.

> PERFECTLY HEALTHY: Wild rice actually isn't rice at all. It comes from a species of grass that produces edible seeds resembling rice. It's also higher in protein and lower in calories and carbohydrates than brown rice or white rice. It's nuttier and chewier than brown rice or other types of rice and is a nutrient-rich addition to your diet.

Per Serving: Calories: 472; Fat: 24g; Carbohydrates: 48g; Fiber: 10g; Protein: 23g; Sodium: 518mg

Roasted Edamame, Veggies, and Walnuts

Dairy-free, Gluten-free, Sheet pan, Vegan
SERVES 4 | **PREP TIME:** 10 minutes | **COOK TIME:** 25 minutes

I love sheet pan dinners where you can just throw away the foil after you're done cooking. This sheet pan meal is a delicious combination of veggies, edamame, and walnuts roasted until tender and then drizzled with a quick Italian dressing. If you've never had edamame before, you are in for a treat. Edamame is the actual soybean—high in protein, fiber, antioxidants, and fiber. You can find it shelled or unshelled in the freezer section of most grocery stores.

FOR THE ROASTED VEGETABLES

Nonstick cooking spray

3 cups baby carrots, quartered (see Substitution Tip)

3 cups green beans, trimmed (see Substitution Tip)

2½ cups frozen shelled edamame

½ cup walnut pieces (see Substitution Tip)

1 tablespoon avocado oil

½ teaspoon sea salt

FOR THE DRESSING

2 tablespoons extra-virgin olive oil

2 tablespoons red wine vinegar

1 teaspoon Dijon mustard

1 garlic clove, minced

½ teaspoon dried oregano

½ teaspoon dried parsley

½ teaspoon sea salt

¼ teaspoon freshly ground black pepper

TO MAKE THE ROASTED VEGETABLES

1. Preheat the oven to 400°F. Line two baking sheets with aluminum foil and spray with nonstick cooking spray.

2. In a medium bowl, toss the carrots, green beans, edamame, and walnuts with the avocado oil and sprinkle with the salt. Transfer the vegetables to the prepared baking sheets and roast for 20 to 25 minutes, until the vegetables are caramelized and soft.

3. While everything is roasting, whisk the olive oil, vinegar, mustard, garlic, oregano, parsley, salt, and pepper in a medium bowl until well combined.

4. Transfer the roasted vegetables to a large serving bowl. Pour on the dressing and mix well. Serve immediately.

> SUBSTITUTION TIP: The great thing about meals like this is that they are very customizable and versatile. I've tried this recipe with many different veggies. My husband's favorite was when I added red bell peppers. Feel free to get adventurous by substituting different vegetables and various types of nuts, but keep the edamame so you get enough protein!

Per Serving: Calories: 402; Fat: 26g; Carbohydrates: 29g; Fiber: 12g; Protein: 18g; Sodium: 419mg

Chile Lime Baked Cod

30 minutes or less, 5-ingredient, Dairy-free, Gluten-free, Nut-free, One pan
SERVES 4 | **PREP TIME:** 5 minutes | **COOK TIME:** 15 minutes

I'm a huge advocate of stocking your pantry with seasoning blends. Sure, you could pull out 15 types of spices every time to make your own blends, but it's easier to pull out just one jar from the cabinet. One that I like to stock up on is chili lime seasoning or fiesta lime seasoning. It makes these cod fillets come to life. I like to serve them with refried beans and cilantro lime cauliflower rice (page 60).

Nonstick
  cooking spray

3 tablespoons chili
  lime or fiesta lime
  seasoning

4 (6-ounce) cod
  fillets

1. Preheat the oven to 400°F. Line a baking sheet with aluminum foil and spray it with nonstick cooking spray.

2. Rub the chili lime seasoning all over the cod fillets and place them on the baking sheet.

3. Bake for 12 to 15 minutes, until the fish is cooked through, light, and flaky or has reached an internal temperature of 145°F. Serve immediately.

COOKING TIP: **Cod stays fresh in the refrigerator for 2 to 3 days. You can freeze it, but some of the texture and flavor will be lost in the freezer. It's best to cook it as soon as possible after you buy it and eat it right away.**

Per Serving: Calories: 189; Fat: 2g; Carbohydrates: 0g; Fiber: 0g; Protein: 41g; Sodium: 125mg

Baked Salmon Meatballs

30 minutes or less, Nut-free, Sheet pan
SERVES 4 | **PREP TIME:** 10 minutes | **COOK TIME:** 20 minutes

These salmon meatballs are made from fresh salmon instead of canned for an unbeatable fresh taste. I love to serve this dish with guacamole and Fresh Homemade Salsa (page 62) for a seafood-inspired fiesta meal.

Nonstick cooking spray

1 pound skinless salmon fillets, cut into chunks

1 cup whole-wheat panko bread crumbs

¼ cup sour cream

1 egg

2 tablespoons chopped fresh cilantro

1 garlic clove, minced

1 teaspoon paprika

½ teaspoon sea salt

¼ teaspoon ground cumin

1. Preheat the oven to 400°F. Line a baking sheet with aluminum foil and spray it with nonstick cooking spray.

2. Put the salmon in a food processor and process until finely chopped. Transfer to a large bowl and add the bread crumbs, sour cream, egg, cilantro, garlic, paprika, salt, and cumin. Stir to combine.

3. Scoop about 2 tablespoons for each meatball and roll the mixture into 16 meatballs. Place on the prepared baking sheet. Bake for 15 to 17 minutes, until the balls are golden brown and crispy.

4. One serving is four salmon meatballs.

> **PERFECTLY HEALTHY:** Salmon is packed with omega-3 fatty acids that fight inflammation. When choosing salmon, it's best to buy wild-caught salmon or farmed salmon from areas known for better farming practices. These fish will have a higher omega-3 content than conventionally farmed fish.

Per Serving: Calories: 319; Fat: 12g; Carbohydrates: 21g; Fiber: 1g; Protein: 28g; Sodium: 589mg

Teriyaki Shrimp

30 minutes or less, Dairy-free, Gluten-free, Nut-free
SERVES 4 | **PREP TIME:** 5 minutes | **COOK TIME:** 20 minutes

Shrimp is the perfect healthy alternative to chicken for this classic dish. If you'd like to make this a fuller meal, add ½ cup of cooked brown rice to each serving.

1 tablespoon avocado oil

1½ pounds medium raw shrimp, deveined

6 cups frozen stir-fry vegetables

½ cup soy sauce or coconut aminos

½ cup orange juice

½ cup water, plus 1 tablespoon

2 tablespoons honey

4 garlic cloves, minced

½ teaspoon ground ginger

1 tablespoon cornstarch

1. In large skillet over medium-high heat, heat the oil. Add the shrimp and cook for 3 to 5 minutes, until fully cooked and pink throughout. Remove from the skillet and set aside.

2. Put the veggies in the same skillet, cover, and cook over medium-high heat for 8 to 10 minutes, until defrosted and soft.

3. In a small pot over medium-high heat, combine the soy sauce, orange juice, ½ cup of water, honey, garlic, and ginger. Bring to a boil.

4. In a small bowl, mix the remaining 1 tablespoon of water and cornstarch. Pour this into the soy sauce mixture and continue to boil until thickened, 3 to 5 minutes.

5. Add the shrimp back to the pan with the veggies, toss with the sauce, and serve immediately.

PERFECTLY HEALTHY: **Shrimp (and eggs) used to be off the table because of their high cholesterol content. Today, the recommendation is that for the majority of people, dietary cholesterol does not raise cholesterol levels in the body, and the American Heart Association removed dietary cholesterol as a nutrient of concern. Other dietary influences, such as saturated fat, refined sugar, and excess calories, have more pronounced impacts.**

Per Serving: Calories: 318; Fat: 4g; Carbohydrates: 29g; Fiber: 4g; Protein: 36g; Sodium: 783mg

Poultry and
Meat Entrées

Spinach Artichoke–Stuffed Chicken Breast

Gluten-free, Nut-free, Sheet pan
SERVES 2 | **PREP TIME:** 10 minutes | **COOK TIME:** 30 minutes

Spinach artichoke dip is my top appetizer pick any day of the week. My hubby and I eat it for dinner sometimes. Since it's not the most calorie-friendly option, in this version I double-stuffed the dip with spinach and artichoke. Then I stuffed it inside a chicken breast. Creamy, cheesy, garlicky goodness in every bite of juicy chicken? Now, that's dinner!

Nonstick cooking spray

2 (8-ounce) boneless, skinless chicken breasts

1 tablespoon avocado oil

2 cups finely chopped baby spinach

1 cup chopped artichoke canned in water and drained

¼ cup ricotta cheese

¼ cup cream cheese

1. Preheat the oven to 375°F. Line a baking sheet with heavy-duty aluminum foil and spray it with nonstick cooking spray.

2. Make a cut lengthwise in each chicken breast to create a deep pocket (don't cut it all the way through). Coat the chicken breasts thoroughly with the avocado oil and set aside.

3. In a medium bowl, mix the spinach, artichoke, ricotta, and cream cheese. Stuff half the ricotta mix into each chicken breast.

4. Transfer the chicken to the baking sheet and bake for 30 minutes, until the chicken reaches an internal temperature of 165°F. Serve immediately.

COOKING TIP: Add whatever veggies you have on hand as a side dish to make this a full meal. You can use leftovers or roast some vegetables along with the chicken. No need to make life complicated!

PERFECTLY HEALTHY: Artichokes are packed with prebiotic fiber, which means the type of fiber in artichokes feeds the good bacteria in your GI tract, encouraging them to stick around, thrive, and help you out with optimal digestion.

Per Serving: Calories: 481; Fat: 23g; Carbohydrates: 8g; Fiber: 6g; Protein: 57g; Sodium: 1,203mg

Creamy Chicken Broccoli Casserole

Gluten-free, Nut-free
SERVES 6 to 8 | **PREP TIME:** 5 minutes | **COOK TIME:** 90 minutes

This recipe takes longer to come together than I typically want to spend cooking, but it's so worth it. It's the ultimate comfort food that everybody loves: juicy chicken, chewy brown rice, and tender broccoli tossed with a velvety-rich, creamy cheese sauce, all topped with a browned cheesy crust. It's not what you think of when you think of healthy, but in this case, it actually is! I lightened up the sauce and added more broccoli than is typically found in your everyday cheesy casserole.

3 cups water

2 cups brown rice
(see Cooking Tip)

1 tablespoon avocado oil

2 pounds boneless, skinless chicken breasts, cut into cubes
(see Cooking Tip)

4 cups broccoli florets
(see Cooking Tip)

3 tablespoons flour

4 cups milk, divided

1 tablespoon butter, melted

2½ cups shredded Cheddar cheese, divided

1 cup plain Greek yogurt

½ teaspoon sea salt

½ teaspoon freshly ground black pepper

½ teaspoon garlic powder

Nonstick cooking spray or avocado oil

1. Put the water and brown rice in a medium saucepan and bring to a boil over medium-high heat. Cover the pan, reduce the heat to medium, and simmer until the liquid has been absorbed, 40 to 45 minutes. Remove from the heat, keep the pan covered, and let the rice sit for about 10 minutes.

2. While the rice is cooking, heat the oil in a large nonstick skillet over medium-high heat. Add the cubed chicken and cook for 15 minutes, until the internal temperature reaches 165°F and no pink remains. Set aside.

3. Fill a medium saucepan halfway with water, insert a steamer, and put in the broccoli. Cover the pan and steam the broccoli for 6 to 8 minutes, until fork-tender. Set aside.

4. In a small bowl, whisk together the flour and ½ cup of milk until completely smooth.

5. Place a medium skillet over medium heat and pour in the melted butter. Add the flour mixture to the skillet, followed by the remaining 3½ cups of milk. Cook and whisk constantly for 7 to 10 minutes, until the sauce mixture is thickened. If the flour begins to stick to the bottom of the pan, remove the pan from the heat for a few seconds, turn down the heat, then set it back on the burner, and continue whisking. You will know your sauce is done when you feel some resistance on your whisk.

6. Turn off the heat but do not remove the pan from the burner. Add 2 cups of the shredded cheese ½ cup at a time, until fully incorporated. Add the yogurt, salt, pepper, and garlic powder and mix until combined.

7. Preheat the oven to 350°F. Spray a 9-by-13-inch casserole dish with nonstick cooking spray.

8. In a large bowl, combine the cooked rice, broccoli, chicken, and creamy sauce. Mix well to combine. Pour the mixture into the casserole dish. Sprinkle with the remaining ½ cup of cheese and bake for 40 to 45 minutes, until the casserole is golden brown and bubbly on top. Serve.

COOKING TIP: **Want this recipe to come together just a tad bit faster? Buy frozen precooked rice or instant brown rice and precut broccoli florets that can steam in the bag. You can even swap the chicken for rotisserie chicken. This will cut the time required for this recipe almost in half!**

Per Serving: Calories: 745; Fat: 36g; Carbohydrates: 51g; Fiber: 3g; Protein: 53g; Sodium: 749mg

Cajun Chicken and Creamy Zucchini Noodles

Gluten-free, Nut-free
SERVES 4 | **PREP TIME:** 10 minutes | **COOK TIME:** 25 minutes

This recipe uses the same seasoning suggested for the blackened cod in week 1 of the meal plan (Blackened Cod and Parmesan Zucchini Slices, page 56), so you can see how versatile spice blends are. If you don't want to invest in a spiralizer right now, that's okay! You can buy pre-spiraled zucchini noodles in many grocery stores in the produce section, near the salad kits and precut veggies.

2 tablespoons Cajun seasoning

¼ teaspoon sea salt

¼ teaspoon freshly ground black pepper

1½ pounds chicken tenders

1 tablespoon avocado oil

¼ cup cream cheese

¼ cup ricotta cheese

½ cup grated Parmesan cheese, divided

¼ cup milk

1½ teaspoons butter

2 garlic cloves, minced

4 zucchini, cut into zucchini noodles

1. On a medium plate, mix the Cajun seasoning, salt, and pepper. Toss the chicken tenders in the seasoning mixture to coat.

2. Heat the oil in a large nonstick skillet over medium-high heat. Pan-fry the chicken, cooking for 10 to 12 minutes, until light golden brown all over, flipping halfway through. Remove the chicken from the skillet and set aside.

3. In a small bowl, mix the cream cheese, ricotta, ¼ cup of Parmesan cheese, and the milk.

4. Melt the butter in the same skillet you used to cook the chicken. Add the garlic and cook for 1 minute. Add the cheese mixture and stir for 1 to 2 minutes, until thickened. Set the sauce aside in a small bowl and rinse the skillet.

5. Heat the clean skillet over medium heat. Cook the zucchini noodles for 3 to 5 minutes, until warmed. Add the cheesy sauce and mix well to coat. If the zucchini starts to give off a lot of water, turn the heat up to high and cook until the sauce is thick again and the water has evaporated, about 10 minutes.

6. Stir in the cooked chicken and the remaining ¼ cup of Parmesan cheese. Serve immediately.

COOKING TIP: **If you feel comfortable multitasking, I suggest mixing the cream sauce and cutting your zucchini into noodles while you wait for the chicken to cook. It will make the whole process much faster.**

Per Serving: Calories: 404; Fat: 19g; Carbohydrates: 11g; Fiber: 2g; Protein: 50g; Sodium: 1,242mg

Lightened-Up Skillet Chicken Pot Pie

Nut-free

SERVES 4 | **PREP TIME:** 10 minutes | **COOK TIME:** 55 minutes

I'm pretty sure that my husband could live on pot pie alone, he loves it so much. The problem is that it's usually very calorie-dense and time-consuming to make. This recipe uses rotisserie chicken, frozen veggies, and a premade whole-wheat pie crust—all measures that save a lot of time without sacrificing any flavor. Mirepoix is a mix of diced celery, onions, and carrots.

⅓ cup all-purpose flour

2 cups 2 percent milk

2 cups chicken broth

½ teaspoon sea salt

½ teaspoon freshly ground black pepper

½ teaspoon dried thyme

2 tablespoons butter

1 russet potato, peeled and diced

2 garlic cloves, minced

2½ cups (10 ounces) frozen mirepoix mix

½ cup frozen peas

½ cup frozen carrots

3 to 4 cups shredded cooked chicken

1 whole-wheat unbaked pie crust

1. Preheat the oven to 375°F. Line a baking sheet with aluminum foil.

2. In a small bowl, whisk together the flour and milk and set aside.

3. Heat a medium saucepan over medium heat. Bring the chicken broth to a boil. Add the flour mixture. Cover the pot with the lid, but remove it every 30 to 60 seconds to whisk the liquid. Continue for 5 minutes, until the sauce is thickened. Mix in the salt, pepper, and thyme. Remove from the heat and set aside.

4. Melt the butter in a cast-iron skillet over medium-high heat. Add the potatoes and garlic. Cook for 5 to 10 minutes, until the potatoes are browned. Then add in the mirepoix mix, peas, and carrots and cook until soft, about 10 minutes.

5. Add the chicken and sauce and mix well to combine. Spread everything out in the skillet and top it with the pie crust. Make several slits in the crust to allow steam to escape.

6. Place the cast-iron skillet on the prepared baking sheet. Bake for 30 minutes, until the pie crust is golden brown. Let cool for 10 minutes before serving.

PERFECTLY HEALTHY: **Many health food stores carry whole-wheat pie crust that's made without preservatives, trans fats, or otherwise sketchy ingredients. Admittedly, they are more readily available at the regular grocery store during the holidays, so I usually stock up then. If I can't find a whole-wheat version, I just buy a regular one that contains clean ingredients.**

Per Serving: Calories: 841; Fat: 45g; Carbohydrates: 75g; Fiber: 15g; Protein: 39g; Sodium: 1,799mg

Creamy Spaghetti Squash Casserole

5-ingredient, Gluten-free, Nut-free
SERVES 4 to 6 | **PREP TIME:** 15 minutes | **COOK TIME:** 35 minutes

Use your favorite sausage in this casserole—sweet Italian, hot Italian, or any other. Sausage is higher in fat, but that's okay; fat helps you feel full and is necessary for proper hormone balance. Since this dish is higher in fat, we will drop the carbs by using spaghetti squash instead of spaghetti.

Nonstick
cooking spray

1 large
spaghetti squash

1 pound pork or turkey
sausage, casings
removed

1 cup half-and-half
(see Substitution Tip)

1 egg, whisked

1 teaspoon garlic
powder

1. Preheat the oven to 400°F. Spray an 8-by-8-inch baking dish with nonstick cooking spray.

2. Make slits all over the spaghetti squash and place it in a microwave-safe bowl. Microwave for 10 minutes, until just fork-tender, rotating every 3 minutes. It can be slightly undercooked because you will bake it later. Let the spaghetti squash stand for 5 minutes to cool.

3. Meanwhile, heat a medium skillet over medium-high heat. Add the sausage and break it up with a wooden spoon. Add the half-and-half and cook until the mixture is just thickened, 3 to 5 minutes.

4. Cut the spaghetti squash in half lengthwise, remove the seeds, and shred the flesh with two forks to get long strands. You should have about 6 cups.

5. In the baking dish, toss the squash with the sausage, egg, and garlic powder. Bake for 30 minutes, until it's fully set on the top and slightly browned.

SUBSTITUTION TIP: **For a dairy-free option, substitute full-fat canned coconut milk for the half-and-half.**

Per Serving: Calories: 502; Fat: 41g; Carbohydrates: 17g; Fiber: 2g; Protein: 18g; Sodium: 1,090mg

Slow Cooker Stuffed Peppers

Gluten-free, Nut-free
SERVES 6 | **PREP TIME:** 10 minutes | **COOK TIME:** 4 hours on high
or 6 to 8 hours on low

These Mexican-inspired slow cooker stuffed peppers are super easy because the slow cooker does all the work for you. You can even prep these the night before and place them in the slow cooker in the morning to have dinner ready when you get home. I love to serve these with my Fresh Homemade Salsa, but you can use a store-bought brand made with clean ingredients and no added sugar.

1 pound 93 percent lean
   ground turkey

1 (15-ounce) can black
   beans, drained
   and rinsed

1 white onion, diced

½ cup shredded sharp
   Cheddar cheese

1 egg

2 garlic cloves, minced

1 tablespoon
   chili powder

1 teaspoon dried basil

6 bell peppers, red
   or green

¼ cup Fresh Homemade
   Salsa (page 62) **or**
   store-bought salsa

1. In a large bowl, mix the turkey, black beans, onion, cheese, egg, garlic, chili powder, and basil until well combined.

2. Slice the tops off the bell peppers and carefully carve out the seeds.

3. Pour the salsa into the bottom of the slow cooker. Fill each pepper with one-sixth of the stuffing and place it in the slow cooker. Cook for 4 hours on high or 6 to 8 hours on low. Serve.

PERFECTLY HEALTHY: Did you know that bell peppers have three times more vitamin C than an orange?

Per Serving: Calories: 273; Fat: 11g; Carbohydrates: 22g; Fiber: 8g; Protein: 24g; Sodium: 206mg

Barbecue Turkey Meatloaf

Dairy-free, Nut-free

SERVES 4 | **PREP TIME:** 10 minutes | **COOK TIME:** 60 minutes, plus 10 minutes to rest

This homemade turkey meatloaf is a lighter spin on a classic American comfort food. It's tender and moist but not mushy, and it's full of smoky barbecue flavor. I like to pair it with the cauliflower mash that tops the Shepherd's Pie Skillet (page 88).

1 tablespoon avocado oil

1 onion, chopped

2 garlic cloves, minced

2 pounds 93 percent lean ground turkey

¾ cup bread crumbs

½ cup low-sugar barbecue sauce, divided

2 eggs

2 tablespoons Worcestershire sauce

1 tablespoon smoked paprika

1 tablespoon Italian seasoning

¼ teaspoon sea salt

¼ teaspoon freshly ground black pepper

1. Preheat the oven to 375°F.

2. Heat the oil in a medium skillet over medium heat. Add the onion and the garlic and sauté until translucent and tender, 1 to 2 minutes.

3. In a large bowl, combine the onion mixture with the turkey, bread crumbs, ¼ cup of barbecue sauce, the eggs, Worcestershire, paprika, Italian seasoning, salt, and pepper.

4. Place the meat mixture in a loaf pan, top with the remaining ¼ cup of barbecue sauce, and bake for 45 to 60 minutes, until the internal temperature reaches 165°F and the meatloaf is completely set and lightly browned on top.

5. Let rest for 10 minutes before serving.

> PERFECTLY HEALTHY: **Choose a low-sugar (or lowest sugar you can find) barbecue sauce (such as Primal Kitchen or something similar) to keep the calories and sugar in check in this recipe.**

Per Serving: Calories: 338; Fat: 17g; Carbohydrates: 13g; Fiber: 1g; Protein: 32g; Sodium: 400mg

Easy Weeknight Picadillo with Plantains

Dairy-free, Gluten-free, Nut-free, One pot
SERVES 4 | **PREP TIME:** 10 minutes | **COOK TIME:** 35 minutes

Picadillo is a delicious traditional Cuban weeknight dinner. I love spicy food, but my husband doesn't, so this recipe is a compromise, with the medium amount of spice. It's perfect for us any night.

3 tablespoons avocado oil, divided

4 garlic cloves, minced

1 yellow onion, chopped

1 medium red bell pepper, seeded and chopped

1 pound 85 percent lean ground beef
(see Substitution Tip)

4 cups chopped romaine lettuce

1 (15-ounce) can diced tomatoes, drained

1 cup beef stock

½ cup pitted and sliced green olives

¼ cup Worcestershire sauce

1 (4-ounce) can tomato sauce

1 teaspoon dried oregano

¼ teaspoon ground cumin

2 slightly green plantains, peeled and sliced into ¼-inch rounds

1. Heat 1 tablespoon of oil in a medium skillet over medium-high heat. Add the garlic and onion and cook for 1 to 2 minutes, until translucent and tender. Add the bell pepper and cook for 1 minute more.

2. Add the beef and cook for 8 to 10 minutes, until no longer pink. Add the lettuce, diced tomatoes, stock, olives, Worcestershire, tomato sauce, oregano, and cumin and simmer for 20 minutes, until thickened.

3. While the picadillo is cooking, heat ½ tablespoon of oil in a medium skillet over medium-high heat. Working in batches and adding ½ tablespoon of oil after each batch, cook the plantains for 3 minutes on each side, or until golden brown. Serve alongside the picadillo.

SUBSTITUTION TIP: **Picadillo is traditionally made with ground beef, but it would work with ground turkey or chicken as well.**

Per Serving: Calories: 511; Fat: 18g; Carbohydrates: 64g; Fiber: 6g; Protein: 29g; Sodium: 867mg

Coconut Ginger Pan-Fried Pork Chops

30 minutes or less, Gluten-free, Nut-free, One pot
SERVES 4 | **PREP TIME:** 5 minutes | **COOK TIME:** 25 minutes

This Thai-inspired creamy coconut sauce complements delicious pork chops and works beautifully with long-grain brown rice and steamed veggies. This recipe makes plenty of flavorful sauce to coat your pork chops and sides.

- **1 tablespoon avocado oil, plus 1 teaspoon**
- **4 (4-ounce) pork chops**
- **2 garlic cloves, minced**
- **½ yellow onion, diced**

- **1 teaspoon ground ginger**
- **¼ cup coconut aminos or soy sauce**
- **1 cup organic light coconut milk**
- **1 tablespoon freshly squeezed lime juice**

- **¼ cup chopped fresh cilantro, for garnish**
- **¼ cup chopped scallions, for garnish**
- **1 teaspoon sesame seeds, for garnish**

1. Heat 1 tablespoon of oil in a large skillet over medium-high heat. Add the pork chops. Cook for 3 to 5 minutes on each side until they're browned but not yet completely cooked. Remove from the pan and set aside.

2. Pour the remaining 1 teaspoon of oil into the same pan. Add the garlic and onion and sauté until the garlic is fragrant and the onion is translucent and tender, about 3 minutes. Add the ginger, coconut aminos, coconut milk, and lime juice; whisk well, and let simmer for 2 minutes.

3. Add the pork chops back to the pan. Cook until the pork chops are cooked through or reach an internal temperature of 145°F, 15 to 20 minutes.

4. Serve garnished with the cilantro, scallions, and sesame seeds.

> PERFECTLY HEALTHY: **Compared to other cuts of pork, pork chops are relatively lean, and they are a good source of protein, B vitamins, zinc, and potassium.**

Per Serving: Calories: 368; Fat: 24g; Carbohydrates: 12g; Fiber: 1g; Protein: 25g; Sodium: 350mg

Desserts

Froyo Bark

Gluten-free, No-cook, Vegetarian
SERVES 10 | **PREP TIME:** 10 minutes | **CHILL TIME:** 4 to 24 hours

This frozen treat is sweet and creamy, with a chewy honey-walnut crust. It's the easiest dessert to make and is a great healthy snack too. I sometimes nosh on this around 3 p.m., when the sweet cravings hit full-force.

2 cups rolled oats

1 cup shelled walnuts

⅓ cup maple syrup

¼ cup coconut oil

1 to 3 tablespoons unsweetened almond milk

2 cups 2 percent plain Greek yogurt
(see Substitution Tip)

1 tablespoon honey

1 teaspoon vanilla extract

2 cups mixed berries

1. Line a baking sheet with parchment paper.

2. In a food processor, pulse the oats, walnuts, maple syrup, and coconut oil until they form a thin paste. If the mixture is too thick, add the almond milk 1 tablespoon at a time to slightly thin it out. Spread the mixture on the prepared baking sheet.

3. In a medium bowl, mix the yogurt with the honey and vanilla. Pour on top of the oat and walnut mixture. Top with the berries. Freeze for 4 to 24 hours, until solid. Serve.

SUBSTITUTION TIP: **You could sub different low-sugar flavors of Greek yogurt for plain. Try blueberry, key lime, or whatever flavor you like.**

Per Serving: Calories: 219; Fat: 13g; Carbohydrates: 21g; Fiber: 2g; Protein: 7g; Sodium: 29mg

Strawberries and Coconut Whip Cream

30 minutes or less, 5-ingredient, Dairy-free, Gluten-free, No-cook, Nut-free, Vegan

SERVES 6 | **PREP TIME:** 10 minutes | **CHILL TIME:** 10 minutes

Sometimes we forget about classic desserts that are easy to make and taste delicious. This dessert is what eat I when I want something just a little sweet but also luxurious. Turbinado sugar, or raw sugar, is minimally processed and still contains some of the natural molasses.

1 (15-ounce) can coconut cream	6 cups strawberries, quartered, divided	6 teaspoons turbinado sugar, divided

1. Chill both a large mixing bowl and the can of coconut cream in the refrigerator for 10 minutes.

2. In the chilled bowl, whip the cold coconut cream with an electric hand mixer for 5 minutes, until light and fluffy.

3. Divide the coconut whipped cream among 6 bowls. Top each with 1 cup of strawberries, sprinkle with 1 teaspoon of turbinado sugar, and serve immediately.

SUBSTITUTION TIP: **It's good to buy fruit that's in season, since it is typically higher in nutrients and lower in cost. Swap your strawberries for pears in the winter and apricots in the spring, and try Barbados cherries in the fall.**

Per Serving: Calories: 328; Fat: 28g; Carbohydrates: 21g; Fiber: 5g; Protein: 4g; Sodium: 5mg

Chocolate Chia Protein Pudding

5-ingredient, Dairy-free, Gluten-free, No-cook, Nut-free, Vegetarian
SERVES 4 | **PREP TIME:** 5 minutes | **CHILL TIME:** 4 hours to overnight

This creamy, delicious pudding has the consistency of rice pudding but a chocolate flavor. It's the perfect sweet treat to help you hit your daily protein goals.

½ **cup milk**

½ **cup unsweetened cocoa powder**

¼ **cup chia seeds** (see Perfectly Healthy note)

¼ **cup maple syrup**

1. Mix the milk, cocoa powder, chia seeds, and maple syrup in a large bowl. Divide the mixture among four containers.

2. Refrigerate the pudding for 4 hours or up to overnight to set. Serve.

PERFECTLY HEALTHY: Chia seeds can be found in almost any store, usually in the baking aisle or with the nuts and seeds. They are, like other seeds mentioned in this book, nutrition powerhouses, packed with omega-3 fatty acids, fiber, and protein, plus they can absorb 12 times their weight in water.

Per Serving: Calories: 152; Fat: 6g; Carbohydrates: 26g; Fiber: 7g; Protein: 5g; Sodium: 19mg

Salted Dark Chocolate Almonds

5-ingredient, Dairy-free, Gluten-free, No-cook, Vegan
SERVES 8 | **PREP TIME:** 3 minutes | **CHILL TIME:** 1 hour

Most "dark chocolate" almonds you can buy at the store are covered with a semisweet or very low percentage of dark chocolate. The higher the percentage, the more bitter the chocolate, but also the more packed it is with antioxidants and heart-healthy polyphenols. Making your own dark chocolate almonds at home means you can use high-quality dark chocolate that is at least 60 percent cacao or greater. Plus, it makes an excellent activity for kids.

5 ounces dark chocolate (60 to 70 percent cacao)

1½ cups whole almonds, raw and unsalted

1 tablespoon coarse sea salt

1. Line a baking sheet with parchment paper.

2. Melt the dark chocolate in a microwave-safe bowl, 30 seconds at a time, stirring between intervals. It will take from 1 to 3 minutes total, depending on your microwave.

3. Stir the whole almonds into the melted chocolate, making sure to coat each one. Remove the chocolate-covered almonds with a fork and place them on the prepared baking sheet. Sprinkle with the coarse salt.

4. Allow the chocolate to harden. You can speed this process up by placing the almonds in the refrigerator. Serve.

> LEFTOVER TIP: I store these in a giant glass container in the freezer. Since they are free of preservatives and artificial ingredients, they will melt if they're kept outside the refrigerator, especially in the summer.

Per Serving: Calories: 256; Fat: 21g; Carbohydrates: 14g; Fiber: 5g; Protein 7g; Sodium: 304mg

Double Chocolate Almond Flour Muffins

Dairy-free, Gluten-free, Vegetarian
SERVES 12 | **PREP TIME:** 10 minutes | **COOK TIME:** 25 minutes

These double chocolate muffins are tender and moist, like a cupcake without frosting. The use of almond flour instead of refined white flour is more filling and better for blood sugar control, which leads to fewer cravings and easier weight loss. Luckily, they still satisfy your chocolate cravings!

Nonstick cooking spray or avocado oil

2½ cups blanched almond flour

¼ cup unsweetened cocoa powder

½ teaspoon baking soda

½ teaspoon baking powder

¼ teaspoon sea salt

½ cup unsweetened applesauce

½ cup maple syrup

2 eggs

1 teaspoon vanilla extract

½ cup chocolate chips

1. Preheat the oven to 350°F. Grease a 12-cup muffin tin with nonstick cooking spray.

2. In a large bowl, mix the almond flour, cocoa powder, baking soda, baking powder, and salt.

3. Add the applesauce, maple syrup, eggs, and vanilla. Beat with a handheld electric mixer until everything is combined. Fold in the chocolate chips.

4. Divide the mixture among the muffin cups and bake for 18 to 24 minutes, until a toothpick inserted in the center of one comes out clean. Serve.

LEFTOVER TIP: **Are you making this just for yourself? Make half a batch or freeze the leftovers. They will keep for up to 3 months.**

Per Serving: Calories: 279; Fat: 16g; Carbohydrates: 32g; Fiber: 5g; Protein: 7g; Sodium: 88mg

Chocolate Chip "Nice" Cream

30 minutes or less, 5-ingredient, Dairy-free, Gluten-free, No-Cook, Vegan
SERVES 4 | **PREP TIME:** 10 minutes

My grad school roommate and I used to make "nice" cream all the time in college. Not that there is anything wrong with ice cream—except that how often two stressed-out nutrition students wanted to consume it could have been a problem. I love this version because it tastes like a creamy chocolate-covered banana (another grad school favorite) in ice cream form. No churning required!

2 cups frozen sliced bananas

⅓ cup cashew butter

½ cup unsweetened vanilla almond milk, divided

2 teaspoons vanilla extract

3 tablespoons mini chocolate chips

1. In a food processor or high-powered blender, combine the banana, cashew butter, ¼ cup of milk, and the vanilla.

2. While the processor is running, slowly add 2 tablespoons of milk at a time, up to another ¼ cup, until a thick, creamy texture is achieved, scraping down the sides as needed. Stop adding milk when you have a thick ice cream texture.

3. Turn off the machine and mix in the chocolate chips. Serve immediately.

LEFTOVER TIP: If you want to freeze this for later use, you can; it will keep about 3 months. When you are ready to eat it, take it out of the freezer and let it defrost for 10 to 15 minutes before digging in.

Per Serving: Calories: 296; Fat: 15g; Carbohydrates: 39g; Fiber: 4g; Protein: 5g; Sodium: 64mg

Caramelized Plantains

30 minutes or less, 5-ingredient, Gluten-free, Nut-free, One pot, Vegetarian
SERVES 3 | **PREP TIME:** 10 minutes

Plantains are a tropical staple and a close cousin of bananas, though they contain more starch. Unlike bananas, plantains are almost always cooked before eating them. The plantains used in an earlier recipe in this book were yellow and not ripe at all, resembling a potato in texture. For this recipe, be sure to use fully ripened plantains—the skin should be almost totally black. They are much sweeter and appropriate for a delicious caramelized dessert.

2 tablespoons
  salted butter

1 teaspoon maple syrup

1 large ripe plantain,
  peeled and cut into
  ¼-inch slices

1½ cups double-churned
  light vanilla ice cream

1. Heat a medium skillet over medium heat. Add the butter and, once melted, stir in the maple syrup. Add the plantain slices and cook for 3 to 5 minutes, until golden brown; then flip and cook them on the other side for another 3 to 5 minutes, until golden brown.

2. Serve with ½ cup of double-churned vanilla ice cream per serving.

> PERFECTLY HEALTHY: **Plantains are similar to bananas but more versatile, and they're nutrient-rich. Just one plantain is a good source of fiber, vitamin C, and potassium.**

Per Serving: Calories: 452; Fat: 24g; Carbohydrates: 44g; Fiber: 2g; Protein: 3g; Sodium: 24mg

Baked Cinnamon Sugar Donuts

30 minutes or less, Nut-free, Vegetarian
SERVES 12 | **PREP TIME:** 15 minutes | **COOK TIME:** 15 minutes

Donuts are such a special treat any day of the week. When I was a kid, I remember looking forward to eating them on weekend mornings or after a dance recital. These donuts taste like the ones I remember but are baked instead of fried, saving tons of calories but preserving the flavor. The cinnamon sugar crust melts in your mouth with every delicious bite.

FOR THE DONUTS
Nonstick cooking spray

1½ cups whole-wheat pastry flour

½ cup coconut sugar

1½ teaspoons baking powder

¾ teaspoon baking soda

¾ teaspoon cinnamon

½ teaspoon salt

½ teaspoon ground nutmeg

¾ cup milk

6 tablespoons salted butter, melted, divided

1 egg

1 tablespoon vanilla extract

FOR THE TOPPING
½ cup granulated sugar

1 to 2 teaspoons cinnamon

TO MAKE THE DONUTS

1. Preheat the oven to 350°F. Spray a 12-hole donut pan with nonstick cooking spray.

2. In a large bowl, mix the pastry flour, coconut sugar, baking powder, baking soda, cinnamon, salt, and nutmeg. Set aside.

3. In a medium bowl, whisk together the milk, 3 tablespoons of melted butter, the egg, and vanilla.

4. Pour the wet ingredients into the dry ingredients and mix until smooth. Put the batter in a large ziptop bag, cut off a bottom corner, and pipe the filling into the donut pan.

5. Bake for 12 to 15 minutes, until a toothpick inserted in the center of one comes out clean. Cool in the pan for about 10 minutes before moving the donuts to a wire rack to cool completely.

TO MAKE THE TOPPING

6. In a small bowl, mix the granulated sugar and cinnamon.

7. Brush the donuts with the remaining 3 tablespoons of melted butter and then dip each into the sugar and cinnamon mixture.

LEFTOVER TIP: **That is, if you manage to have leftovers, you can store them in the refrigerator for up to 1 week. I doubt they will last that long though!**

Per Serving: Calories: 173; Fat: 7g; Carbohydrates: 26g; Fiber: 2g; Protein: 3g; Sodium: 153mg

MEASUREMENT CONVERSIONS

Volume Equivalents	U.S. Standard	U.S. Standard (ounces)	Metric (approximate)
Liquid	2 tablespoons	1 fl. oz.	30 mL
	¼ cup	2 fl. oz.	60 mL
	½ cup	4 fl. oz.	120 mL
	1 cup	8 fl. oz.	240 mL
	1½ cups	12 fl. oz.	355 mL
	2 cups or 1 pint	16 fl. oz.	475 mL
	4 cups or 1 quart	32 fl. oz.	1 L
	1 gallon	128 fl. oz.	4 L
Dry	⅛ teaspoon	—	0.5 mL
	¼ teaspoon	—	1 mL
	½ teaspoon	—	2 mL
	¾ teaspoon	—	4 mL
	1 teaspoon	—	5 mL
	1 tablespoon	—	15 mL
	¼ cup	—	59 mL
	⅓ cup	—	79 mL
	½ cup	—	118 mL
	⅔ cup	—	156 mL
	¾ cup	—	177 mL
	1 cup	—	235 mL
	2 cups or 1 pint	—	475 mL
	3 cups	—	700 mL
	4 cups or 1 quart	—	1 L
	½ gallon	—	2 L
	1 gallon	—	4 L

Oven Temperatures

Fahrenheit	Celsius (approximate)
250°F	120°C
300°F	150°C
325°F	165°C
350°F	180°C
375°F	190°C
400°F	200°C
425°F	220°C
450°F	230°C

Weight Equivalents

U.S. Standard	Metric (approximate)
½ ounce	15 g
1 ounce	30 g
2 ounces	60 g
4 ounces	115 g
8 ounces	225 g
12 ounces	340 g
16 ounces or 1 pound	455 g

RESOURCES

These resources are ones I regularly share with my clients and recommend often.

Websites and Blogs

American Heart Association (heart.org/en/healthy-living/healthy-eating/eat-smart/nutrition-basics/mediterranean-diet): A guide to the Mediterranean diet—a healthy way to eat and maintain weight loss

Choose My Plate (choosemyplate.gov): Up-to-date information on portion sizes from the U.S. Department of Agriculture

Egg Nutrition Center (eggnutritioncenter.org): Nutrition facts and great recipes for eggs

Environmental Working Group (ewg.org/foodnews/dirty-dozen.php): The latest information on fruits and veggies with highest and lowest levels of pesticides

Healthy People (healthypeople.gov): Up-to-date nutrition guidelines from the Office of Disease Prevention and Health Promotion

Hungry Hobby (hungryhobby.net): You can find additional resources such as nutrition guides, workouts, recipes, and meal plans on my blog

National Resources Defense Council (nrdc.org/sites/default/files/walletcard.pdf): A full list of mercury levels in different types of seafood

Produce for Better Health Foundation (fruitsandveggies.org): Nutrition, storage and handling information, and recipes for a wide variety of fruits and vegetables

Apps

Aaptiv Fitness (aaptiv.com): I use this app for workouts and love it

Cronometer (cronometer.com): Track meals and fitness and health data

EWG Healthy Living (ewg.org /apps): From the Environmental Working Group, includes the latest information on toxic substances in produce, cleaning products, and skin care

Nike Training Club (nike.com /ntc-app): I've used this app for workouts and loved it

Books

Amer, Chelsey, MS RDN, CDN. *The 28-Day Pescatarian Meal Plan and Cookbook: Your Guide to Jump-Starting a Healthier Lifestyle* (Emeryville, CA: Rockridge Press, 2020).

Amidor, Toby, MS, RD, CDN. *Smart Meal Prep for Beginners: Recipes and Weekly Plans for Healthy, Ready-to-Go Meals* (Emeryville, CA: Rockridge Press, 2018).

Gellman, Abbie, MS, RD, CDN. *The Mediterranean DASH Diet Cookbook: Lower Your Blood Pressure and Improve Your Health* (Emeryville, CA: Rockridge Press, 2019).

Shallal, Kelli, MPH, RD, CPT. *Meal Prep for Weight Loss: Weekly Plans and Recipes to Lose Weight the Healthy Way* (Emeryville, CA: Rockridge Press, 2019).

REFERENCES

Chainani-Wu, Nita. "Safety and Anti-Inflammatory Activity of Curcumin: A Component of Turmeric (*Curcuma longa*)." *The Journal of Alternative and Complementary Medicine* 9, no. 1 (2003): 161–68.

Kaipainen, K., C. R. Payne, and B. Wansink, "Mindless Eating Challenge: Retention, Weight Outcomes, and Barriers for Changes in a Public Web-Based Healthy Eating and Weight Loss Program." *Journal of Medical Internet Research* 14, no. 6 (2012): e168.

Lin, Bo-Wen, et al. "Effects of Anthocyanins on the Prevention and Treatment of Cancer." *British Journal of Pharmacology* 174, no. 11 (2017): 1226–43.

McLoughlin, Rebecca F., et al. "Short-Chain Fatty Acids, Prebiotics, Synbiotics, and Systemic Inflammation: A Systematic Review and Meta-Analysis." *The American Journal of Clinical Nutrition* 106, no. 3 (2017): 930–45.

Menon, Venugopal P., and Adluri Ram Sudheer. "Antioxidant and Anti-Inflammatory Properties of Curcumin." In *The Molecular Targets and Therapeutic Uses of Curcumin in Health and Disease,* 105–125. Boston, MA: Springer, 2007.

Thompson, Janice J., Melinda Manore, and Linda Vaughan. *The Science of Nutrition*. 4th ed., Hoboken, NJ: Pearson, 2016.

Turrini, Eleonora, Lorenzo Ferruzzi, and Carmela Fimognari. "Possible Effects of Dietary Anthocyanins on Diabetes and Insulin Resistance." *Current Drug Targets* 18, no. 6 (2017): 629–40.

Yamaguchi, Taichi, Kojiro Ishii, Masanori Yamanaka, and Kazunori Yasuda. "Acute Effect of Static Stretching on Power Output during Concentric Dynamic Constant External Resistance Leg Extension." *The Journal of Strength and Conditioning Research* 20, no. 4 (2006): 804–810.

Yu, Ting, et al. "Effects of Prebiotics and Synbiotics on Functional Constipation." *The American Journal of the Medical Sciences* 353, no. 3 (2017): 282–92.

Zhu, Yongjian, et al. "The Effect of Anthocyanins on Blood Pressure: A PRISMA-Compliant Meta-Analysis of Randomized Clinical Trials." *Medicine* 95, no. 15 (2016): e3380.

INDEX

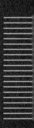

ACKNOWLEDGMENTS

I FIRST WANT TO THANK GOD BECAUSE WITHOUT GOD, NONE of this would be possible.

I want to thank my husband, affectionately known to my blog readers as Mr. Hungry, for supporting me in every way possible, including prepping ingredients as my sous chef and doing endless dishes while I tested recipes for this book.

It would be irresponsible not to mention the state of affairs, as we were in the beginning of the coronavirus pandemic when I did the bulk of writing this book and testing the recipes. I want to thank my nutrition clients and blog readers for asking for the resources they needed to get back on track after their lives had been turned upside down by COVID-19. Many of them asked for a full guide, including a 30-day meal plan and workout information, and I'm so grateful for the opportunity to provide that for them and for everyone who reads this book.

ABOUT THE AUTHOR

KELLI SHALLAL, MPH, RD, CPT, CLT, is a registered dietitian in private practice with a master's degree in public health from Loma Linda University and a National Academy of Sports Medicine certified personal trainer. She is the author behind the popular healthy living blog *Hungry Hobby* (HungryHobby.net) and the owner of healthy meal planning company What to Eat? Meal Plans. Her first book, *Meal Prep for Weight Loss,* is ranked in the Top 100 for Mediterranean Cooking, Food & Wine; Weight Loss Recipes; and Weight Loss Diets on Amazon. Kelli's advice and recipes have been featured in major media outlets, including *Today's Dietitian, Food & Nutrition Magazine, Good Morning Arizona* (3TV), AZTV, *Shape, Fitness Magazine, Health, Runner's World, U.S. News*, and *Self.*

Kelli lives in Phoenix, Arizona, with her husband, Paul; young son, Kal; Rhodesian ridgeback pup, Nala; and cat, Missy. Find out more about Kelli on her healthy living blog HungryHobby.net, and follow her social media @hungryhobby (Facebook, Pinterest, Twitter) and @hungryhobbyRD on Instagram.